When The Fog Lifts

One Woman's Journey

Through Multiple Concussions

and Fog-lifting Messages of HOPE!

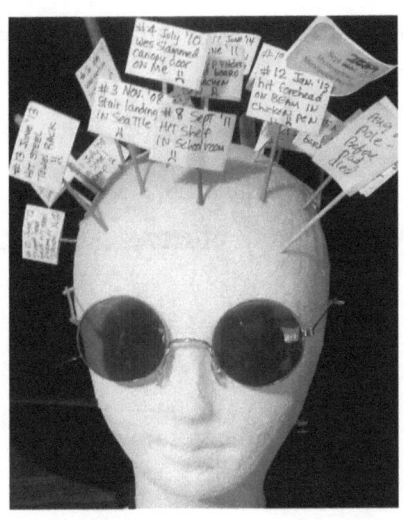

LAURIE LEE LEWIS

This book is dedicated to *YOU*.

The one who is brave enough to look at life's FOG...

face it, walk into it and have the courage to lift it!

I pray this book brings hope, understanding about brain injury and all types

of fog that can roll in − to teach, to serve and help us grow along the way.

To suggest that fog might be a teacher.

To all the hearts that have tried to understand my journey and
love me through it. Thank you!

***

To my GIFT FROM GOD "Daughtie" my Callieflower -

Callie Anne Lewis. *I love thee ever so.*

Thank you for being born and choosing me to be your mom.

***

*To **mom**, thank you for caring for dad through all of the fog and,*
being the reason I got the gift to write songs and poems!

***

For those who thought I made this up, well maybe this book will help
you understand, and should you or a loved one ever travel this road,
maybe a few of my words will bring you encouragement and hope.

For teaching me to live with a gentle, heart-centered life;
encouraged me to sing loud and proud, and sit up tall in the saddle,
taught me some **very** unique vocabulary, that makes the angels laugh,
like how to give a damn and not give a damn,
and who truly knew his little Lollee's heart...
My favorite cowboy! Ride on, **dad**, ride on... High In The Saddle.
This book was finished in memory of my dad, Jack J. Little.

Content:

Special note:

This book took 10 years to live and write - for you, and for me.

So what I want to say right here, right now is...

If this is an actual paper book, and not borrowed from a friend or library, I encourage you to underline, highlight, right in notes.

Make it your book. Your fog lifting commitment ... to you!

I am not an author. Or a teacher... but I am. So are you!

I do not do things perfectly. I just write.

A friend once said that she was ALL about editing, editing, editing! My reply politely was, "I am all about living, living, living, and then writing. Editing last!"

So my hopeful pearls of wisdom might be sandwiched in a story, poem OR a goofy expression that I learned from my dad, like: HORSE SHIT!

So PLEASE... come along with me on this fog lifting ride. You might get saddle sores trying to understand my country gal jargon, but hang in there. Watch out for low hanging branches!

If I can grow food to feed the masses from my beautiful dirt, I ought to be able to share some tidbits about FOG.

HUGS and GIDDY-UP!

love, Laurie

The Story Behind The TITLE

I printed out an editing copy of this book in February 2019, to see how I did with my layout and such. Bloopers. Bleeps and Blunders! It is a hefty enough read - without that stuff, but boy oh boy, it was pretty funny!

You will be surprised after you read this, just how many people use the word FOG to describe miserable or painful, unclear places in their life. But, you may also hear remarkable stories of when their fog lifted.

I pray my attempt here will help lift some of yours too, if it is hovering over your life right now.

This book would not have this title without the following story. While it is not concussion-related it IS a very foggy story.   I wanted you to read how long I have been saying: WHEN THE FOG LIFTS.

In March of 1996, 2 years before my daughter was born, I found myself on an airplane coming home from Maui. Sounds fun, don't it? I was sitting by a beautiful, elderly Asian woman with broken English.   When we hit the air, she looked at me, my depleted, sad soul, and said, *"You look like you have quite a story."* I replied softly, *"Oh, I do."*

With her gentle encouragement, over the next few hours I unfolded the story. I told her that I had fallen in love with a married, but separated man, over a year prior. Such a powerful relationship, but his wife would not grant him a divorce and instead moved with their 2 little boys to Montana. He was devastated. But loved me and was so torn. So was I.

With a weird twist of fate, I happened to find an ad, that a entrepreneur in Maui had place, and was looking for a few key people to help him finish his recording studio and spiritual retreat.   How this could be, was beyond me.   I contacted him. Told him that I came from both of those backgrounds and would love to be part of this magic.   He shared that there was a cabin on the land and the studio construction had already begun. I believed him. I *needed* to.

I suddenly knew that in order to do the "right thing" I needed to move away, disappear, and send the man I loved to Montana - to be with his children, even if the marriage could not be restored.

23 years from the day of writing this, in early February 1996, I sold everything I owned, found a home for my dog,Willy, (which was brutal) and bought a ticket to Maui. I was to leave late February. My heart was busting, but I knew this was what I had to do.

The day before my flight, I went to a clinic because stress had apparently made the menstrual cycle stop for January/ February and I had some ovary pain.   Hard to forget this day, when the nurse came bounding into the room with good news, "You are pregnant!"

Telling my love about this, the night before flying out, was horrible. He begged me to stay. So many tears. My guts were in knots.   He was clear he would stay. Talk about tempting to a tender heart.   Instead, I had him drive me to Seattle and I boarded the plane to the unknown, carrying his baby, weeping most of the flight, as I had let go. Not the most painful day of my life, but certainly painful to a pregnant girl who loved a boy.

The shortest possible version of this story is, the man in Maui (Lani) turned out to be a scammer, drug-using, liar. I got there and I was instantly stuck. The cabin was a shack that leaked. I slept in a tiny cubby full of spiders. There was no bathroom. There were 2 men plus the coming and going owner.

I was terrified, but decided to play calm and cool because the other was too brutal. Too potentially panic-strickening.

This guy, Lani, did have the land. It was fairly magical. Undeveloped. It was Maui after all. But not one construction thing started! Only in his head and on paper! Oh, wait, I think there was a post in the ground! Studio! Ha! I was sad, scared, lost. Beyond fogged in. And, there was barely any food! Miles from a store. And, no fresh water. Just a garbage can with a screen to catch rain water. HONESTLY! Woohoo!

Ironically, I felt pretty safe and grateful because of the 2 other young men. They were just there for the adventure, total gentlemen and soon learned I was pregnant. While it is a nightmare story, but huge blessings were waiting. *"Please continue"* said to the woman on the plane. So I did.

Over the next couple weeks, we worked. I cried a lot at night. We did some clearing on the land with a lot of heavy lifting. Lani showing up now and then. There was NO money. No budget. It all seemed surreal. But we were there, making the best of it. I prayed a lot. Something so huge, how could this end?

One afternoon, lifting pallet boards, I suddenly began cramping and spotting. Of course no bathroom and bleeding. The guys put up a curtain outside with a bucket that became the elegant commode for the lady! I knew I had made this choice, so tried not to complain, but the spotting and cramps scared me.

The next day, Lani arrived very agitated acting. He and I headed toward town to do laundry. En-route we nearly got ran off the road by a mad driver. We suddenly stopped and a guy got out and was screaming at Lani. Threatening him. When Lani got in I nervously asked what it was about. Turns out we were driving an *unpaid for* van! *THAT* was the owner! Furious! He gave Lani one more day to pay and left. Lani was suddenly a different guy. I went quiet. The road was twisty and he seemed to jerk the corners. I began to feel so sick.

Getting closer to the town, I finally spoke up and said I was not feeling very good. Suddenly, Lani went goofy. Maybe drugs, maybe the stress/guilt. Or both. He began yelling at me and pounding on the steering wheel about me showing up pregnant. He missed his turn so he quickly pulled in to a circle turn around at the Pukalani Mall. As he slowed on the corner something told me to get out. I opened the van door and jumped out tripping, then ran to the mall and did not look back. Heart racing.

All my belongings and what little savings I had - were in his shack, in my dinky cubby. No cell phones back then! All I had was a backpack with dirty clothes and a few dollars.

The Asian woman on the plane reached over and grabbed my cold hand, holding it gently, leaning in to me, she asked me sweetly, *"What did you do, dear girl?"*

I got in the mall, found a restroom, bought supplies from a vending machine, shocked and shaking. By then, I was bleeding fairly heavily. I sat down on the bathroom floor and cried. Gathering my composure, I went back in the mall. It seemed like a different world. I found a phone booth and made a painful collect call home to WA state to tell my folks that things might go badly. That I loved em. I had lied on the calls before, saying everything was fine. My sweet dad offered to sell his tractor to bring me home. I balled.

Eventually I found a security officer and asked about a shelter for the night. I was so dazed and felt ill and hungry. He said he would try to help me if I could not find help by 10 PM., closing. Talk about fog and freaked out.

This is going somewhere, I promise. The title of the book!

10

I felt so alone.   I walked a bit in the mall, following a long wing, where I began to smell ... cookies! I was so hungry. It was late afternoon and I had not eaten since the day before.   In my state of mind, I think I thought I was going to bleed to death or miscarry, and this would be my karma for loving a married man.

I continued toward the aroma, rounded the corner to find: Ms. Field's Cookies!   Something made me go in and decide that if I was going to die or penniless, my last meal was going to be: a cookie and coffee!

The most beautiful, angelic face suddenly appeared at the counter asking if she could help me. What a loaded question! I put the few dollars on the counter. I am sure I must have looked very pale, puffy-eyed and spaced out. Standing there in my little shorts, hiking boots and a backpack.

I asked her what my, I think $2.50 would buy.   She frowned a bit, then and asked if I was okay.   I went silent. Then looking into her coal black eyes, black long hair in a pony tail and the most incredibly beautiful Polynesian face, tears began to well up. I told her that I had just baled from a van, was in trouble, and maybe miscarrying. Immediately, her eyes filled with tears.

She pointed to a table for me to go sit down. She brought me a cookie and coffee. Her hand touched my shoulder as I sat there, still shaking and thanked her. I ate and sipped slowly. I had no place to go. No rush. I had no intention of sharing my story. But it happened. I felt numb.

She disappeared in the back for a little while, then silently again she appeared by my table and said, "My name is Leilani and you are coming home with me!" "What?" My eyes widening with tears.   She said, "I went in the back, spoke to my son, and prayed. God told me to bring you home with me."

The lovely Asian woman - could not believe this story,

squeezing my hand softly, moving in closer, her shoulder touching mine. I continued...

This woman, Leilani, took me to her home. A single mom with 4 boys. Tiny little house. She let me sleep. Cry. Talk. Eat. Prayed with, and for me.   I laid down a lot and the bleeding slowed. She even took me to a clinic, showing that I was still pregnant.

I stayed with her for several days. We bonded like sisters. On about the 5th night, around 2 A.M., I quietly got up feeling very strange. I reached in the fridge, got and opened a yogurt – when all the sudden I got a huge cramp, and a large amount of blood came out. I doubled over with pain, yogurt hitting the floor. Somehow, Leilani was instantly there and helping. I could not believe how she knew.   Within minutes, her eldest son was carrying me to her van and we went to ER.

Over the next 8 hours, Leilani held my hand in ER as my body sent me through hell. Contractions that were huge. Bleeding. They would not medicate.   Finally at 10 A.M. an ultrasound confirmed that I had miscarried.   Leilani took my exhausted self home and cared for me. I cannot describe the next 24 hours. Loss on top of loss, on top of shock.

I got a hold of a dear friend from Canada. Told her what happened. She wired money for me to get a ticket to fly back to Seattle, which, put me on that plane, with that Asian woman, in that moment.

To this day, I believe I owe my life to Leilani. A true angel. When I told her that, she surprised me with: "No Laurie, YOU are the angel. I do all this praying with God, thinking I am being a good Christian, but only now have I really used it." Thanking me!

The lovely Asian woman squeezed my hand again, looking at me shaking her head.

The plane finally landed. I was so exhausted and so sad to be coming home to nothing. No dog. No man. No stuff.

Fractured dreams. FOG. Nothing. My love had followed my wishes and moved to Montana. I wanted no contact.

We all got up, grabbed our over-head luggage and I managed a smile to this sweet woman. She reached out and touched my shoulder and said, *"Laurie, you should write a book."* I reached and touched her shoulder right back and said, *"Maybe someday,* **WHEN THE FOG LIFTS***!"* Then thanked her for listening. We walked off of the plane in silence.

As we walked into the boarding/un-boarding area, she came back up to me and softly whispered as we parted ways, *"Laurie,* **WHEN THE FOG LIFTS** *will be the title of your book."* Gave me the softest hug then walked away. I held back tears.

That was over 23 years ago. MANY chapters of life have followed. In and out of fog. My daughter arrived in my arms 2 years later! My greatest gift God has given me.

All of this, 12 years before my first concussion in 2008.

HERE I AM. Who'da thunk! Okay, let's do this.

WHEN THE FOG LIFTS

PREFACE

To you who *actually* read the Preface. Hmm, Pre-face. Interesting. My description or question of that word would be: what or who is behind the face?

How do you write a book about brain injuries, when you are the brain injuries? Someone once said to me, "Laurie, you AREN'T your injuries. YOU were injured, but don't let it own you." That is shop talk for: YOU ARE WHAT YOU THINK. I get it. I understand. I believe it. But, when your thinker of thoughts... gets *thonked*, and fog moves in, well, life changes. Those folk with their clear thoughts can easily say that. Cuz there thinker is thinking!

Reality, spiritualizing and/or mind-power thinking, are great. But in the moment, when we are barely functioning, adding another responsible or accountable thought about our injury - can make things worse. It can feel like they are trying to speed us up to bust through the other side.

Authors make bazillions off of their new find, youtubes, downloads, videos, books, and now coaching programs, convincing you that you NEED them. Funny thing is, if we aren't careful in our vulnerable foggy state, we can place our whole future into another person's hands and wallet. Reality, we do not live their lives. We don't see them on a day to day basis. Practicing what they preach! While I have heard successful stories and outcomes from all of this, I have also read, how some went bankrupt, had a nervous break down, divorced, spiraled, some 10 years later after "success!"

So I am not going to tell you, read this sucker and baboomba... your fog will lift forever. I don't live your life. You don't live mine. It is what I have seen my whole life in HOW we decide to use fog and this life, whatever shape we are in, that seems to be the shifting for our lives and growth.

Over spiritualizing - well, instead of embracing the experience of injury, fog, death, loss, ... the new way seems to say YOU created this. YOU attracted it. Deal with it! Get over it! Get on with life. Hmmm. This sounds less compassionate, less caring, less loving energy, to me. That is not cellular healing. In fact, if we aren't careful, GUILT can walk in and start chewin' on de ass. Like we need fog and ass chewin'!

Going back to my friend's words of: "You are NOT your injury." Well, when you wake up almost everyday, not sure if fog will be present or not, and stacked with multiple head injuries, (not hang-overs) well, that one is hard to nod to your friend, agreeing, and saying, "Of course, of course, it is my mind that thinks I had brain injuries. What was I thinking!" Hmmm!

Since 2008, tallying up over 20 head bonkies to heal from – finding clarity, reflection and SURVIVING has been no small task, let alone, trying to share it. Not all concussions, but re-hits on top of hits. Lotsa fog, lotsa blessings.

Furthermore, how do you convince a reader to trust that any of these words are true accounts of an accident? Or many? I have always marveled at this question. Because, I know, we each perceive an experience differently. Some of us go into the victim mentality that asks, "Why me?" While others say, "Okay, bring it on!" Kinda depending on how you view life: as school - or this fleeting blink of time to get all ya can. Or... a bit of both.

Writing WHEN THE FOG LIFTS, has been one of the longest and biggest challenges to date. As a songwriter, starting at 8 years old, and throughout my whole life, I learned to tell a story, idea or emotion in about 3 and ½ minutes. The length of a song. One page. So to write a book and speak at length about healing from injury and challenges - has stretched me beyond measure.

Besides letting you into my world, I am taking off the mask of *I am fine* - to let you see something. Not polished. Not professional. Although I do declare I can say, I did have a 10-year career as a professional head bonker! Unpaid. No endorsements though! I proclaim: *that I am done with this type of experience* and feel clear enough to have gleaned some important pearls of wisdom to share with you here.

I have shuttered a few times in deciding to share this story, and believe me, convinced myself that someone else could do it better or my journey isn't unique enough to share. I am not a boxer, skier, bull rider, football, soccer or hockey player. Just a simple country singing farmer. So how does someone end up hitting their head so many times since 2008?

I look back and grin with the fact that I can type. I speak without stuttering, unless you interrupt me over and over. I have gotten on a plane a few times in the past couple years. I can sing songs again. Remember most lyrics. I drive. I can dance again without falling over, most of the time. I can go listen to music now and then. I have been my folks' caregiver. (Now that - is a good one: brain-injured caregiver!) Ha! I do not have seizure episodes anymore. I am learning to trust myself. Value my precious head and life! Wow! And, through this fog lifting: *opening* to my self-worth.

So, to you, the brain and heart reading this – you may be the injured one. Or married to the injured one. You may be the ex or possibly one considering romantically loving the injured/healing one. You may be the parent, sibling, child, caregiver or friend.

I pray that I can share my journey with you – authentically. There are many levels and layers to this journey. I hope to be taken back to experiences with clear head and open heart. To maybe bring you a little comfort, insight and HOPE to say, "DON'T GIVE UP!"

Other than spell check, this book is as-is. Like buying a car. "As-Is". There is no doctor. No pill. No consultant or copy and paste from the internet to write this puppy. This is my heart to you and a message worth sharing. My PRE-FACE.

One lil extra thangy:

As a child, my dad's nickname for me was Lol or Lollee. I remained that until about 18. In my soul I have leprechaun DNA, I think. So most everything I have gone through, no matter how foggy, I have reached for the silver lining. Maybe not while in the fog, but eventually. I certainly have been to the edge several times. But eventually I would be shown a blessing.

I want to leave this page and start this book with 4 ancient, handed-down, from generation to generation, pearls-of-wisdom, by **ALL** the leprechaun family circles:

1. What goes around, comes around.
2. The Magic is in You!
3. You make your own luck
4. Life is the rainbow, love is the pot of gold!
(You may quote me!)

May this book, in its un-conventional-*ness*, help you see that at the end of the day, *lifting fog*, we have much more power than we think. But, we have to deal with the ooee gooey spaghetti stuff, between our ears first.

Have you ever had the flu? Surgery? Divorce? Miscarriage? Abortion? Depression? Lost a loved one? Car accident? Audited? Lost your job? Spent time in jail? Moved? Went bankrupt? Took cold medicines that wiped you out? Been stoned or drunk? Been dumped? Flunked an important test? Recipient of gossip? Lost your wallet? Got robbed? House burned down? Heart Attack? Cancer? Got in an abusive relationship? Menopause? An affair? Hysterectomy? Felt controlled by a church or another person? Just to ask a few.

Or how 'bout this, you go to town, have a lovely evening, begin driving home and suddenly you cannot see the road 5" in front of you. The fog is so thick. Suddenly you have to dim your lights, slow your car way down, and hope and pray that no one rear ends you or you smash into someone, or a deer jumps out, or you drive through a stop light. When you finally get home, both relief and exhaustion take over. Whew! Fog.

There. I just told you what it is like to have a concussion. LIFE deals you FOG. In the fog you are forced to slow down, pull over, your lights are on dim. You may have to stop. You CANNOT see what is coming next. It can be exhausting. How will you survive? Fear enters. Sorrow. Belief. Faith.

Everything gets scrambled from the reality you knew just before you got the call, accident, loss of job, marriage, loved one or - hit your head. But nearly every foggy story I have ever heard or experienced, had that silver lining, and something else happens.

The stories, if we truly listen and share, begin to connect us to each other. It begins to crack open a place inside of us that was closed. Asleep. A deeper meaning awakening. We all know some type of fog. Some might consider it punishment. Some say it was the greatest thing that ever happened to them, eventually.

The things listed above, generally have a healing time. Some can actually be understood by cause and effect. Your own actions. Or life being life. Brain injury can be that too, the difference is - it is your computer. It is the thinker of your thoughts. Your processor of what is happening. Your hopes, strengths, highs and lows. Rationalizing. Judging. Understanding. Sleep. Hormones, Memory. Physical abilities.

The brain does it all, and when the hard drive just got scrambled with no back-up, we are in trouble. Basically, passwords don't even work- because healing can be sideways. For many, we are never the same. We are changed. What we change and grow into is the challenge for all of us, from life's journey.

What good could possibly come from fog? If you look back at your life every time fog rolled in, what came of it?

This book is going to tell you my story of how a scrawny, singing, organic farmer managed to thump my noggin' many times. Which, in reality, isn't a big deal. Many of us hit our heads plenty. It isn't about the many times. It is about the one that changes everything, and for me, the ones that followed after.

I write this book with no idea if I will still be here by the time you read it. None of us know that. I hope so. I'd like to think I will get to hear someone say, "Your words brought me hope, Laurie." But who knows. I marvel at the fact that each morning I do wake up and get another day. Can't say that about some of the days going through this journey, but THIS DAY - I give thanks!

You will not, with each word I have typed, have any idea if I had a migraine. Blurred vision. Ears ringing loudly. Spell check saying, "What the hell did she type?" On quite a few of my words. Because you get the finished product. You will not have seen me struggle to recap from notes to share this. You will not be able to see how my eyes would swell after a hit, face go numb etc... So it is my attempt to let go of the anxiety that wants to show up from writing and remembering – to push through and share.

You see, being a smiley soul, full of amazement that I get another day – people often have a hard time believing ANY of this happened to me.   Truth be told, MOST of the list of FOGS in the first paragraph of the Preface - have happened to me.   That's a lot. A *lotta* fog. And I am still here. Thanking "my version" of God, everyday!

This I know - as I prepare to share over a 10-year journey with you – this life is not finished until I take my last breath and exit this ol' scar-filled skull and book off to my next journey. As much as I wanted to chicken-out to write this book, maybe this wacky sharing will bring hope.

On chicken, what also helped me be brave enough to write this, was when I went looking at the library for books on concussions and Dementia, most were technically too advanced for me to read. I remembered once hearing Jack Canfield, founder of *Chicken Soup for the Soul®* books, say: *"If you can't find the book you are looking for, then maybe that means you are supposed to write it yourself."* Thank you Jack!

Also as I type, I hope the heck I hit the save button, back it up, and NOT drop my computer!   Basically, that is a damn good visual of hitting your head. Pick up your computer if you have one, and drop it. See what happens when you try to open it up. (Kidding!)

Okay, deep breath in, Laurie. You can do this. It's TIME. Let's write.

Fog, fog, you little hog,
You block my view ahead.
I cannot see - in front of me,
my heart-rate's up - with dread.

I ask for help - as I drive through,
on my road of life -
To slow myself down, and honor the fog -
and try not to fear - this strife.

Please show me fog - what I am to learn,
then lift me and help me grow -
to write this book with seeds of hope,
and love as I type and sow.

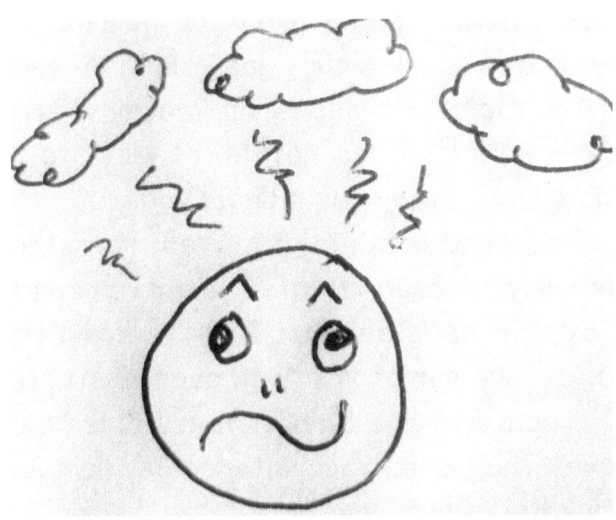

Chapter 1 - TIME

Time and change. The two guarantees in life. Some spiritual leaders say time does not exist. We are ever-lasting. We simply shift to spirit energy or recycle, *or* head off to heaven for everlasting life. Others treat this life as the last. Try to do your best. Obviously *something* is happening to my once tight and perky skin (bet you thought I was gonna say boobs, didn't ya) and my naturally brownish-red hair. Yes, all natural, no grays. No. Bahahaha!

  If we live long enough, while we start out knowing "nothin'" we get to grow and evolve through everything that happens to us. Then, depending on the journey, some might believe they knew it all along, just had to remember. Of course if brutal Dementia shows up, we may just leave this world as we came in, knowing "nothin" at least to the outsider looking in. So I say: "Enjoy the ride as you go!"

  So - TIME and brain injury. Well, now, that's a funny one.   The only reason that I can remember detailed information of thumps is because I wrote down the thumpies, best I could, before symptoms took over. I stuffed my notes in a bag and prepared for a bumpy ride. I tried to jot exactly what happened that day, that altered my life and sent me down the black hole - over and over.

  Even I am amazed that I did this, cuz I am NOT organized. I did not want to but, if I hadn't written it down I could not be writing this book.

Plain and simple: I would *NOT* want to remember that TIME. Suddenly from happy home-school mama and wife to a vege-brain. Dropping and crawling on the floor when my balance attacked me. Finding myself starring aimlessly out in my gardens with a hoe in my hand, not sure what to do next or how I got there. Asking my little daughter or hubby, "What did I just say?" No, I was very happy to forget all of that!

Aside from brain thumps, it is a lot, just keeping up with life. Going through ginormous things like big moves, a divorce. A hysterectomy. With the bonks, when asked to perform my music, fear to commit was right there, because time was warped. But, on the flip, I was inspired to write and produce many songs and CDs for charity and other humanitarian projects. All while under the influence of Post-concussions.

Forgive me here, but reading that back, I have just been *hit* with an all-encompassing expression. HOLY SHITKIES! Disclosure: There might be a few more Laurie-isms ahead. Maybe not suitable for grade-schoolers.

Hitting your head - you may either lose or gain humor. My humor has returned. I have experienced both. On this journey, I could watch a hilarious show and stare straight at it, emotionless - to nearly peeing my pants laughing so hard at the littlest things. Dare I say, at one point, even dating a lovely professional stand-up comedian, I found myself one beat ahead of him firing out jokes - that I made up on the spot! It is a wild ride.

By the time you are done reading this book, you will wonder if I am actually living in a mental facility with a pretty lil' white straight jacket and meds and writing this through my shrink! HEHE. Nope. Right here, down on the farm!

This is me. Singing farmer Laurie. From heaven-on-earth, Northwest Washington state. My sanctuary farm. At my home-made long farm table that I built from old boards (cuz, well, I needed a table.) SO - I built one.

I hope I can show the wildness and potential of turning our noodle thumps into something magnificent. Profound Pasta! The wonderful lemons into lemonade. Over-cooked spuds into mashed taters!   Mmmm. Mmmm.

By the way – I am honored that you are reading this. I care about you.   So I wanted to share something here. I just read that if you are slouching or holding this writing low on your lap, tipping your head forward is like **60 pounds** of weight on your neck! It is suggested to lift your book, phone, reading device to eye level.   I try, but my arms get sore!   I am learning to prop up books or dig a hole to sit in! Ha!

Also, I hope you will read, stop, stretch, drink water, move your spine, take a vacation, in between chapters. Writing this puppy, I figured that part out quickly: writing is an unhealthy posture! Too much sitting. So, I turned it into a challenge. Write. Stop. Vacuum. Write. Stop, eat. Write. Stop. Plant a whole farm. Write. Stop, let a month go by or almost chicken-out of writing it at all. Then, start writing again. Giving myself TIME to do this - the best I can.

If TIME is an illusion, I have often wondered if concussion was too. My brain disagrees. Wonder if I created this to alter my way of seeing life. Too caught up in the past, the future and even the now of bills, family drama, emotions that drained me and enhance my insecurities. By hitting my head, altering those brain waves, I was forced to shift.   To realize, okay, this was my new reality.   Shoot, there were times, I could not bend and tie my shoes without falling over. I could not drive. Or process fast talking, know-it-alls. Or life-bitchers. I avoided them. I hid. Psst, shhhh, don't tell, but... sometimes, I still do!

When you have a brain injury you find out that we live in a bit of a rude society! Or – we don't, but it may appear that way to the struggling, altered mind. Or, as Forrest Gump said,

"I think it is a bit of both."

So if TIME is an illusion, why couldn't I fast forward the injuries and get back to what I was doing just before I bonked? TIME also was in my face day after day, having to start over every morning – FOG as thick as snot. A morning amnesia. Balance off. Tipping over walking down the halls. Acquiring more black and blue elbows.

One would have thought I had a viciously abusive marriage from the bruises I wore - just trying to walk a straight line. (Just for the record, my daughter's daddy was a rock. He knew my stuff, and I will always be grateful regardless, of a divorce.) Going through those thumper puppies, carrying the load as single mom, and helping my folks... while healing, *that* was rough.

As I type this, I am noting my heart rate going up a bit. Remembering. Remembering the sense of being worthless. A burden. My daughter's eyes. The disappointments due to my limitation. Not able to go to concerts, movies, the fair, city, busy streets, trying to walk the speed of others, lights, carpet smells, blaring bass speakers, more than one person talking to me, the mall... and on and on.

When in the fog, sometimes wishing God would just take me home, so my daughter and then, husband could deal with that part and get on with finding a really cool, healthy-brained woman, they could laugh with. (Very sad memories.)

And then I discovered something new about TIME. Which, I am proof of, at this moment of typing, (should include here for your entertainment) that I could NOT type after several bonkies. I became dyslexic. For a long time. I humored several friends who later said, "Yes Laurie, it was often a struggle to read your emails!" Well something beautiful happened - because of TIME... slowly – even with reoccurring hits - I have healed the big issues. TIME is medicine!

Some things, like loss of a loved-one – TIME almost stands still. Feeling like you will never heal. Grief and loss are fogs that can last a very long time. It thins and thickens, begins to lift, then socks back in. But as we know, from incredible people that have lost someone, then turned that grief and loss into a mission to help others, actually helped them heal as well. Helped them live a purpose-directed life.

Pain can be so deep. The work to heal from pain and even having the *time* to do so, while keeping up with life – can be over-whelming. Somehow, however, giving yourself TIME is critical. Otherwise, it can come back and bite later.

Our society is pretty sucky about grief, loss, injury. We are in this *hurry-up,* or - *this doesn't work with my schedule* or *my view of you"* world.   Losing the person you were before brain injury and then trying to live in the new you – has so many layers.

So when family or friends do not know what to do with this NEW YOU, and sometimes, it seems, they accidentally or on purpose, forget to call. Or stop by. TIME for them, can feel like a few days - yet to you, a year could pass by.   On the other hand, you may be glad they stay away. As I did. I did not want them to see me altered. Suffering. Staggering. Barely getting through days.   I would wait til the fog would lift at least 50% before I would even venture out.

But for most of the other FOGGY issues, TIME is amazing. Just look back. Look at anything you have gone through.   When FOG was so thick you never believed you would get through that divorce, cheating spouse, over-drawn account, surgery, post-pardon blues, test, school, job, illness, those lonely nights, whatever...   TIME was the medicine.

So, you or your loved one went kerbonk or stroke or ? Suddenly personality, energy, posture, communication, emotions are strangely altered.   Suddenly there is the awareness of either NO FILTERS or mega FILTERS on what comes next. Meaning, some personalities bust through like steroids with an altered brain, that either become very shut down, recluse, quiet - or unstoppable. Ballsy. Fearless. Because the brain has a fog of reality covering: *balance*. I know this well.

With some of the hits, I would recluse. Afraid to talk because I could not keep up or would stutter. I was the quiet one. Other times it was like, what the hell, and I would blurt things out that I never would say otherwise. In fact, it opened a door to stand up for myself to some key people in my life that had enjoyed some viscous back-stabbing. Suddenly I was pushed to a place that said, "You know what? NO MORE!"

Or suddenly I would hug someone and tell 'em I loved 'em. An act that I may have held back before. I think I felt as if I would heal from this someday, and forget what I went through. So I HAD to do things. Like TIME was critical. Or, I would get worse and wanted to leave behind: love.

The bad thing on this is that a bruised brain may not want to go to sleep because of TIME. The reality that it may have taken the whole day to regain enough cognitive thinking to do something. So by nighttime, why go to sleep and have to start over in the morning? (Oh my gosh, thank goodness for spell check) I wish you could have seen all the red marks on these pages before I cleaned them up!

By the way, I rarely put a "g" on the ends of my words. Or they come and go. So you can imagine spell check's frustration with this lil country gal's verbiage. It will actually put the g on words when I am not looking - to make me sound extra intelligent or something! Woohoo!

I want to leave two things in this writing about TIME.
1) I have a tremendously difficult time with TIME. Schedules can bring anxiety. Appointments, details too close together. Oddly, I have done things like big

concerts, meetings, producing projects and about 2 to 3 weeks later - I can awaken, and completely think I have to *go do* those things. This is improving, but sometimes it makes me wonder how present I was during a concert. During producing. At a meeting. But I sure try.

Since I am doing my best each day, I do not beat myself up over this as much anymore. Thought maybe I was TIME *traveling*. This part of me is getting better. But as I have shared with others - my biggest fear, being single most of the past 6 years, has been that I would give my heart to another and one day ... wake up and ask, "WHO ARE YOU?" YYYYYOUCH! More on that later...

2) The 2nd thing I am learning is: to try not to get *stuck* in and *on* TIME. Because life has proven over and over we go through and come out of fog, changed. Even if just a tiny bit.

When the fog lifts... we have an opportunity to see a new piece of our unlimited potential selves. WHEW! Time ... for coffee!

Oh you bugger -
that ticks away,
telling me, "wake up -
or be late today."

Raising my blood pressure -
if I get behind,
I have no use for you -
obnoxious time.

~

Except of course -
if it brings a day,
where I can relax -
create and play.

Wull dang... I think -
I'll make this rhyme,
and have more days -
like that - with time.
LLL

Chapter 2 - Hope

HOPE. Man, now there is a powerful four-letter word, along with LOVE. What would we do without them? I will talk about love later... right now, where and however this finds you in your life, perhaps reaching through fog and pain for HOPE - for you, or someone you love.

- ⅄ Hope is what has gotten me out of bed in the morning.
- ⅄ Hope is what has told me to go ahead an order seeds for my spring planting.
- ⅄ Hope is what inspired me to write, record and release music CDs to help humanity.
- ⅄ Hope is what I have held on to and HOPED that the things I taught my daughter would be enough to help her through her own life, especially if I wasn't here.
- ⅄ Hope is where I placed my faith, when family and friends have misunderstood me over the years, hoping someday, they would take the time to know the real me.
- ⅄ Hope is what I drew off of when I hit the darkest of dark. Wanting to leave this life. Feeling like a burden.
- ⅄ Hope is what I held when I lowered my guard to try to love again.
- ⅄ Hope is what I hold as I type these words for you and me.

With hundreds of rejection letters from publishers and record labels during my 30-year music career, I admit my HOPE waned. Finally resorting to recording my own songs and releasing on my own little label. Seeing minimal sales and spending lots of money. The illusions to others that I was rakin' in the dough was hard. Instead, I was struggling. But HOPE has been the calling forth to glean from all of this and keep on, keepin' on!

Today, this modern social networking age, super stars are everywhere. But in my generation, if you came in a pretty decent package, big smile, tall and thin, and dared to dream, well, right there, you might subject for judgment. The, "who does she think she is" stuff.   Then get older or injured and continue trying... it is hard for some folk to understand. Man, I get it.   To try to sing and hope to remember words, shaking with nerves and not giving up. It is a big deal. It is easy to quit. Except when the call, calls you, again.

Perhaps that is why I love being a farm girl. My critters don't judge. I can show up butt ugly, bad breath, swelled eyes and they love me. Or dolled up. I look the same to them.

HOPE is that beautiful whisper to: *HOLD ON... when darkness walks in. HOLD ON... and let go of what others think.   With brain injury, HOPE is all you have at times, because time may disappear, while in the fog.*

When the fog was heavy from bonk 3 or 4, and I was trying to walk down to the barn to check on goats and horses. I was struggling severely to take steps.   I walked like a duck. My motor skills were altered.   I often used a little stick for balance. I remember thinking over and over, "what if I stay like this?   Thank goodness no one can see me walking today. Thank heavens I have the farm and can hide during this time." I would weep. My coordination stunk. If I held more than 2 items in my hands, I would get anxious. If more than one person would talk at me, I would shake. If someone talked too long and I could not track, I wanted to cry or escape.

All I had during those times, was HOPE. This wasn't like my surgeries on my foot or insides. That, I understood. That took TIME. Medicine. Therapy. HOPE was that teeny little seed... waiting under the soil for the right moment to germinate and pop through the FOG. Farmers know a lot about hope. For sun, soil, long days, water, good crops etc. and each season can change. HOPE sits there to fall against and catch us ... when we rock backward to far and say, "I DON'T KNOW IF I CAN DO THIS."

Where I have found HOPE living in me, which might sound weird - but is in the one thing most of us can have some awareness and control of: breath. A deep breath in, realizing whatever I am doing, about to do, will most likely not kill me. But bring me an experience in life. Letting out the breath of relief. WOW. When I figured this out, it really pushed on the fog bank. I swear it has helped lift some of the thickness and anxiety many times. But of course, I am no pro - I will certainly forget this information too, and probably need to read this chapter!

HOPE seems to be tied in with GRACE. It tells you that you cannot control life. Life is happening. But you can insert your intentions ... to say: I AM getting better everyday. I WILL walk straighter. Talk clearer. Type again. Sing again. Dance again. Love again. I will - because I believe. I have HOPE. In fact, HOPE can be your dearest companion. Even worth naming her or him as a little sweet guardian angel up there fluttering in your noggin, helping you! To call on and is always there. Okay, yes, starting to sound like a Pixar movie!

Funny how HELP and HOPE start with h end with a p... sound. See what you too can come up with by scrambling your eggs up there between your ears? A whole new way a thinkin'!

The fun part of writing this book - that has been started and tossed about 10 times over 10 years... is some knowing that I could not write until significant TIME, ah time, had passed. I mean really, who would want to read it, if I was stuck in the fog. Sheesh-ka-bobbles!

The other benefit to not being a scholarly type brain, with no medical background, is I get to share with you as THE BRAIN - meaning I may jump around. Share a story when you least saw it coming or sing you a little ditty.   YELL OUT "THANK YOU GOD" practicing another medicine: *gratitude*.

I think I have some big surprises in the pages that follow. Hopefully you will laugh and *feel*. For when we feel, we identify, even if each others pain comes from different experiences. Loss is loss. A healing heart and mind need time, hope and love and the more we can learn, the more compassion and grace we can have.   Bonking my brain busted open my heart.   Bringing me here! Can you see me waving at you?

I have a lil story about HOPE that I believe is well-worth sharing at this point. In desperation, I sought out help. Prepare yourself. Sit up and take note. THIS IS CRITICAL!

This story starts with a blue oval rug.

In Spring 2015, I found myself and then, 15-year-old daughter - alone. Marriage had fallen apart. In trying to fix up my old house, I saw a blue oval rug for sale on Craigslist. Met the gal, paid for the rug and got talkin' about our lives. Told her, back then, I was on a rough batting average and had over a dozen bonks. Some hefty, some light - but still symptomatic.

I told her how I felt like my marriage died because my screwed up brain finally gave up trying to live with an intelligent man, who had shifted from religious to atheist during our marriage. Which was okay, because it seemed to broaden his view on life, but being a spiritual chickie... I clung harder to my faith and hope - that I would heal.

As I shared my story the woman's eyes widened. She said, "You *need* to go get assessed for disability, Laurie. You cannot possibly hold a job, support yourself, daughter and farm, injured." I disagreed with her about the disability. Said I did not have any interest in receiving money for my brain bonks. It did not feel ethically right and I would find away to survive and was receiving some support from soon-to-be ex.

She understood but went in and got me a number for a neurologist, that is considered one of the most renowned doctors in the Northwest. For respect and to not get my lil ass sued, I shall refer to him as Dr. J. (Lol, I first typed "sewed"! Oh dear!) The woman suggested I go get assessed anyway. Because, she could see in my depleted, depressed spirit, that I had lost a lot of hope, and felt maybe I was going nuts!

The big oval rug was perfect for our living room. I kept the number, and finally got gutsy enough to call it. The very idea of talking about this stuff bugged me. I had already seen a doc twice about some seizures I had- with one of the hits. She made me feel like I was making it up. So "above" me in her persona and title. AKA: Me, peon with head bonk, her big chief with degree - on de wall!

I remembered questioning my condition after talking to that doc. So to do this again, yipe! But, a little voice said this might give me HOPE. Because right then, and on and off over 7 years, my ex and young daughter had gone through hell and probably would at least like to know I did this.

I got an appointment. Had to wait over a month. Finally the day came to go see this powerful OZ of brain injury and, wouldn't cha know it, I had a migraine. Oooh doggies. Big one. Eyes were puffed. Balance off. Light sensitive. Ears ringing. Really had no business driving. But I was determined.

I had purchased some hay from a man a few weeks before this - who told me his ex-wife had gone through a bad concussion and an assessment. When I told him I wanted to do it, he warned me, "They don't always turn out the way you want them to, Laurie." Gulp.

I arrived 15 minutes early. Had already filled out pages of my information at home. My head really off. But I got to thinkin, "Well, maybe this will be okay. Rather than be in good shape, right?" As-is.

Walking to the office, taking an elevator up, then just getting down the hallway, my eyes started spazzing out at the wild line patterns on the carpet. Thinking, now *there is a seizure maker!* Got in the office and ended up sitting for another 30 minutes past my appointment time. By now I was wishing I had brought a protein bar and Excederin. My blood sugar was feeling a little wonky. I kept thinking, "Laurie, you got yourself here. He is a specialist. He will help give you back hope and dignity. Hang in there, girl."

Finally a receptionist came out and got me. Put me in an office facing a big window. Oops. This was going to get worse. My eyes don't do well looking into light. Especially with a headache already going. I looked down and closed my eyes. Door opened. In walked a slender, tall man, with a bearded-face and long pony tail. First thought, *woohoo*, he looks organically cool and hip. Nice! He reached out to shake my hand. His hand shake was cold and wimpy but hey, I am a farmer. Lotsa wimpy hand shakes out there! But - no judging.

Dr. J told me that the appointment would be approximately 3 hours. With a battery of test for different parts of the brain. Long and short recall, cognitive, comprehension. Oh boy. About then a young handsome man walked in and also shook my hand, introduced himself, and said he would be assisting on this test because it was part of him becoming a neurologist. I thought, cool. He seemed nice, good eye contact, and I felt a kindness from him. Not so much from Dr. J.

Dr. J went over my papers and said he had looked at my

recent MRI. Agreed that I had a lot of white marks of scar tissue all over my noggin'. So I think we had established bonks had happened. (HATE THEM MRI's) 4 in 8 years. PLENTY. Yuck yuck and yuck!

To bring validity and a little humor to my appointment, I brought something in to show the doc. Now, you might get by now, that while some folk get big owees (or little ones) I try not to be of the victim mentality. More survivor-thriver. But I have met plenty of people that only focus on their ailments, not the blessings.

So, here I was, now about to go into this ass-ess-ment... which would take on a new spelling and meaning after 3 long hours - but won't blow the punchline here.

I pulled out a big styrofoam head from my tote bag and sat it on the desk. She was wearing cool purple sunglasses. In which I considered borrowing, in this piss-poorly-lit office - facing a window! Both men looked a little surprised (to say the least.) After-all, hells bells, this is my brain, my appointment, that I waited over a month for, paying $275 out-of-pocket so, I was bringin' my daggum HEAD! "This is THUMPER" I told them.

On the head, were little toothpicks holding tiny signs. Each sign (14, then, I think) had a date and place of each hit, poked in on my skull where I bonked. To an on-looker for the first time, they probably felt like they were looking at a porcupine with sunglasses! The intern smiled, and said, "Cool, I like this."

Dr. J. showed no expression looking at the head, other then turning to me, to say, "Yes, well, lets get started." As he sat down to face me with his back to the window. I said, "I may have to move. I am not feeling very good today and facing windows can mess with me big time." His reply was to last as long as I could. *Geez.* I glanced around for a garbage can, in case I had to hurl.

He glanced through my paperwork that documented all the medications I had tried, MRI appointments, dates, symptoms, my interests, vitamins... everything. As he thumbed through, he noticed the word "seizures." He asked me about them. He noticed and commented that I had seen his colleague, twice, Ms. Dr. T. of this exclusive brainyology club.

First question: "You say you had seizures, following one of your hits to the back of your head. What made you think it was a seizure?" I proceeded to tell him where I hit and how I came up under a 2 x 12 beam, rang my clock, and how within the same day, my face went numb and I began seeing triple. Could not walk. Legs would lock up and could last 1-4 minutes and I was exhausted after. Brain doing a zappy thing. They were happening every few hours for weeks.

When I got in to see Dr. T, she did not believe me. I asked her if she would look cross-eyed as hard as she could, and try to walk. Her dignity and expertise told me she did not need to do such a thing. She prescribed Gabapentin and sent me away. It actually worked if I got to them in time. But, these "episode" dudes continued for 6 months. I did not drive for 5 of them. Did not want to risk a wreck.

Mr. J's response: "Hmmmm." Continuing, he brought up a piece of paper. Said he was going to read 12 words. He wanted me to remember them. I did my best to repeat them when he was done. Then he read 12 more. Again I did my best. Got most of them. He went on to bring out a drawing that was nothing. Doodle scribbled on a page. He wanted me to look at it. Stare. DEEPLY. Then he took it away. He asked me more questions.

By now, blood sugar and head weren't feeling very happy. And that damn window was awful. I asked if I could angle my chair. Or he could pull a shade? No on the shade. Yes on slight angle. Grrrrrr. "You turd" was my inside thoughts!

The intern sat quietly watching the master do his thing, typing notes on a laptop. I did tell Dr. J in the beginning, that I was not here for disability testing, rather, HOPE. With a divorce coming, life was not easy right now. HOPE would be good.

Dr. J suddenly hit me with a curve ball. "Laurie, what were the first 12 words I told you?" Ah... huh? Blank. "Okay, how about the next set of 12?" I got a few. Then he handed me a blank piece of paper and said, "Now draw what you saw of that drawing I showed you." OMGosh! All I could see was a 2-year-old's scribbles. So I just doodled something. "Hmmm" was his profound reaction.

He stood up, and told me his intern was going to take over now. He was leaving. Ah, okay? I think. Nice cute intern sat down with a gracious smile and said he had a lot of questions to ask me. No tricks. Just yes and no. I had to stop many times and shake my head. I needed water. Closing my eyes when he left. He was cool.

Maybe a half hour went by, and in came Dr. J. They switched seats. He pulled out a wooden board with 3 dowels sticking up. Then put rings on the far right one. From small to big on top. Told me to sit there and make all the rings re-stack properly by using both other dowels. This made me start shaking inside. I think he was checking his email, as I tried.

I told him straight out that my mind could not see this type of information. Could we skip it? He said no. I tried and tried. And within maybe 5-8 minutes I felt like I was going to vomit and cry. I dropped my head and said, "I AM SORRY. I cannot do this." He took it away. Asked me those dang 12 words again of group one and two. I think the intern felt bad. I could feel his energy shifting in the room. Like something wasn't right. I sensed maybe Dr. J. wanted me to have a seizure so he could mark it in his book.

We took a little break. Then I was taken to a tiny room with a chair and computer. This was more like a closet. Just big enough to sit in and very stuffy.

Dr. J said, "You will be asked 300 questions. It will be: always, never or maybe - and probably take an hour." All I could think was how would I stay in that dinky room? But I was determined to get a clean-bill-of-HOPE to share with my ex and daughter. It meant everything to me.

The questions were weird. Simple and then stuff like "How often have you pondered killing someone?" Eeeks! Or "How often have you considered sexual pleasures with children?" Oh My Gosh! These made my stomach turn. NEVER button was hit a lot! Then it got to deep darkness. "How often have you wanted to commit suicide?" What? How do you answer that honestly, with ALWAYS, NEVER, MAYBE? Who wrote this retarded thing?

The stuffy room was getting to me. I kept going. Several times, it asked about murdering someone or pedophile actions. With blood sugar, headache, stuffy room and stupid questions - I was losing it. Finally questions 299 and 300 were ridiculous but easy. I opened the door and the receptionist said to go out to the lobby and wait. So I did. Suddenly feeling very alone.

The intern came out and took me back to Dr. J's window-lit office. This time I turned away from the window and got to look at the intern against a wall. Dr. J. came in. Flipping charts. Standing by his intern, proceeded to tell me that he would analyze the computer testing and send me a report. I replied, "Okay?"

Waiting for some cool stuff for him to tell me. He came back with, "Well Laurie, my intern and I have talked about your condition and while we think you perhaps have had some mild concussions, we are not convinced that you had seizures, and not sure these were actual concussions. I turned ice cold.

He continued, "The papers you filled out said you have been taking Ginko Biloba, NAC, Fish Oil and other herbs/vitamins. That you tried a couple of anti-depressants and said they did not help and gave you headaches. You also went through a hysterectomy and instant menopause. And going through a divorce. And that you do music. I am wondering why you don't just get out and sing?" My ice cold - went to heart beating *YOU IDOT* boiling, but I held back.

I shared as best and briefly as I could, that I have written hundreds of songs. Yes, I toured years ago. Yes I have several CDs out. NO I cannot play music right now because my hands/brain won't let me... you asshole." Okay I left those two words off. But dang it felt good to type them right here. Grrrr.

I collected my swirling thoughts and said, "Okay, so you are telling me my hell has not been concussions, even though I listed and pointed to every hit. Not by joy, but because Dr. T, (his compadre of de brain club) the first neurologist, told me to always tell someone when I hit and write it down. Because your brain can swell within 8-12 hours after and kill you." He agreed. I continued, "So you are saying this is menopause, and my 6 months of hellacious triple-cross vision and unable to walk, getting stuck outside, in barns, in the house... weren't real?"

Dr. J paused then said, "I can see you are aggravated." Now, I am for the most part - a lady, but at this point I smiled and said, "NO SHIT." He continued, "We see that you are pro-natural healing and not open to pharmaceutical drugs that I am quite sure could help you heal."

I was so stunned, I took a step forward into Dr. J's space. Put out my hand. Gesturing for a handshake. He met my hand. I said, "Dr. J, I did not come here for disability, I came here for HOPE. Hope, that I was not losing my mind.

Just experiencing an injured one.   You have told me in so many words that you do not believe me.   As if I am lying. What you stand to gain from this is beyond me.   I will say this, I imagine, maybe 30 years ago, when you were an intern, before all the accolades, awards etc... that you came into this field with heart and compassion to help people. But I do not sense ANY of that from you now. Thank you for your time. And wasting mine."

I squeezed his hand as hard as I could with my lil farmer piss-off hands! Then put out my hand to the intern, and said, "You, don't forget this day. I am an honest person who came here seeking hope over a terrible, life-altering condition. You were a pleasure in this horrible day." then left.

It was all I could do to leave that office without busting. Shaking profusely. Mind not tracking. Felt some where between a seizure coming and going to pass out on that frickin' swirly-patterned carpet hallway, to get to the elevator. My vision was getting blurry, but I got to the car. I could barely see the key hole to unlock the door.

When I got in, tears burst forth and flew from my eyes. I swear they hit the windshield.   I cried so hard. Sat there for a long time. Was I crazy? Was he an ass hole? What was that? And then, how was I going to get home? All because I went to buy a blue oval rug.   But can you see why this piece is critical?

I broke out in a sweat writing this one. One person on this foggy brain-injured path can really mess you up.   I will say this, because of this experience with a brainyologist, I got angry and when an opportunity knocked, I stepped way out of my comfort zone enough to do something that challenged my wellness. I learned all about TBI. Traumatic Brain Injury.

HOPE and TIME are huge medicines when you are healing. Finding the right help is the trick!

I know more than finished writing this chapter, when I came across the actual letter that I sat down and wrote to Dr. J following our "session" and mailed to him. I believe I received an email following to say, "I am sorry you did not find the experience helpful."

I thought you might appreciate reading it. It is karmically cool. While our brain may be healing, if we can speak, our words are valuable teachers for each other, and especially to DOCTORS! First, a lil poem:

Dr. J, Dr. J,

Today you took my hope away.

Your diagnosis left me on fire,

with anger because I felt like a liar.

I suffered through - over 3 hours with you.

You got paid for what you do.

Damn to knowledge - but not of heart,

I was honest right from the start.

May our visit disturb your brain.

Just enough - to feel my pain.

And from this day compassion will rule,

your scholarly self - cuz we need you too.

LLL

Here is the letter I sent to Dr. J on behalf of all us foggy brains who experienced an appointment like mine.

Chapter 2 ½   The Letter

March 2013

Dear Dr. J,

If someone would have told me that I was going to spend $275 of my living expenses and almost 4 hours to be asked words, draw a photo, list names and animals, and do a dowel puzzle that I would never do before I had brain injuries, and, walk in with my honest heart to share a 5 year journey to hell and back, only to be told I never had a concussion, those were not seizures and most of this was contributed to menopause, I am pretty sure I would have not gone. Please note that when our time was done, it was me reaching out to shake the professionals hands, to try to say thank you.

Did it ever occur to you that I made this attempt, to give me hope? Did you give me hope? No. You made me feel like I was wrong about something YOU did not experience. And honestly until you do, and find you aren't smart, you can't function and someone makes you feel like you were wrong, you WILL NOT understand. Sad for you, because it would help your empathy. Einstein said "may our technology never surpass our humanity" I realize what he was speaking about today on a different level.

Your hefty 300-some questions in the tiny booth on the computer lending themselves mostly to drug addicted patients, asked me if I was angry or suicidal. How ironic that leaving your office shaking and crying very hard, I felt such anger for trying so hard to answer as well as I could, when feeling so poorly. I felt as if I was back in Dr. T's office as she minimized my symptoms, telling me that I was not experiencing what I thought. Hmm, I guess she crawled on the floor, fell over, stuttered, went cross-eyed and got lost too.

Leaving your office today made me realize I do have to write the book. Not for the brainy doc. That can take some little tests and assess everything about you, but for the person who wonders if they will ever return fully without living on drugs to bring them up or take them down, or sideways. I know that I will start my book with the experience I had with you today. To show the in-personable system to expect - when you do reach out to what you called "Western medicine". I will forewarn families that tests can immediately make you feel stupid and validate how you already feel inadequate. And that I do not recommend them unless you are solely seeking a disability. For if you have pulled and struggled your way back to trying to function, a day like today can set you a hell of a long way backward.

The most beautiful part of my head injuries has been opening up my compassion level to others. Being able to hear their hearts. Listen with my own, not my ego. Remind them that life is a gift. Perhaps that is what you started out in the field to do as well. But to leave someone with the words you said to me, in an already vulnerable place should not go unmentioned. To say I should not use the word "seizures" I think you were trying to protect me from losing my license. To whom? What if I had one and had not mentioned it to anyone?
I asked you for some pamphlets or information on symptoms from areas of the brain. If nothing more than to understand.

I also asked for the phone number of the TBI group person in Bellingham. What did you give me exactly? You walk a fine line in someone's life. I am sure you are aware of this. If I would not have questioned and disagreed - your eyes would never have widened to "Oh this woman does have a voice". Like I said, until you travel to hell and back or part way back, with a brain injury, you only know from how you perceive it. While I do not wish this on anyone, I will speak from knowing and trying to help others. And, to remind people to be aware of their thoughts, they might be the last ones you get! Thank you for this experience. Something I can share.

Sincerely,
Laurie Lewis

I want to add something here:

If you have experienced an appointment such as I did, please, take the time, ballsy up, complain. Or have someone complain for you. This medical world verses actual patient world is VERY screwed up. We know it. No one pays us to endure the hell of brain injury. We aren't blaming anyone. But we deserve extreme respect, for without us - they would not have the profession they get paid for! Heftily, I might add.

So use yours or your loved-ones injury to help balance out this screwy medical world. SPEAK OUT. It isn't like you can get fired! Docs have a tendency to have ups-menship over patients. They cannot fix us, but they have NO RIGHT to belittle or generically diagnosis us. Let's keep them growing too! BE A VOICE FOR US ALL! Not all docs are going to give you this experience. There are incredible neurologists out there as well. It can take months to get in to them, but they are out there. Seek references.

Speak up! Speak up!
For those who have no voice.
We are in this thing together -
advocating is a choice.

Let doctors know that this is real,
and fog is a scary thing–
help them learn – not write us off,
we're a force of reckoning.

Be persistent in finding help,
you're a teacher through it all.
The doctors learn more by treating us
than their degree hanging on the wall!

Chapter 3 - TBI

After my not-impressed and hopeless experience with Dr J. the neurologist, I returned home pretty depleted. I did not want to even talk about the 3-4 hour goofy assessment. In which I broke that word apart and found ass-essment and it made me at least chuckle.

Honestly, I don't swear all that much, but for some reason, writing these memories, I have a little attitude about how some medical folk look down on the injured one. Like we intentionally rattled our noggins for attention or excuse to check out mentally. Quite the opposite. I would not wish the FOG on anyone, but in reality, a little brain rattle to a few of these know-it-all docs, might give them back some empathy, humility and not just a big pay check and accolades.

Well, as life tries to help you... I remember the doctors saying TBI instead of concussion several times. Something made me look up TBI (Traumatic Brain Injury) to research more of what is available to us. I never thought of my concussions as such a dramatic description, but as I read, there are various levels and pretty much all concussions end up under this category. Multiple injuries like mine, get very, very complicated.

Today, research has added a new title to a condition that can result from multiple injuries called (CTE) Chronic Traumatic Encephalopathy, a degenerative brain disease from a history of repetitive brain trauma. Often this can develop years after the traumas. This one made me sit up. Talk about needing HOPE. After you read this book, you will understand why I say that!

The Will Smith movie: Concussion®, was incredibly hard for me to watch, alone.   I wept. Partially because I watched it while still fogged-in. Afraid this time, from hit, like 15, that the fog may not lift.   My life seemed to be shrinking. I could not function out there in our busy, fast, loud world.

In researching multiple concussions, feeling like my story was so wimpy in comparison to a star athlete on TV talking with a stutter, or learning about football players committing suicide to *stop the noise*. But a calling forth said, "Keep writing, Laurie. I too, have a story. I represent the OTHER brains." Sports, for lack of better words and tacky punchlines, is a no-brainer. As I said earlier, drop your lap top some, 10 - 20 times in a year or two, or even once, your hard-drive is toast! So why do we think we can smash, crash, and bash the precious computer on our shoulders and come out fine and dandy?

While there are many online TBI websites now available with wonderful information, I did not find as much on **multiple concussions**. Then, one day researching symptoms of CTE, as I watched my dad's brain rapidly decline in 5 years, going from multiple hits, to stroke to Dementia, and concerned about my own future, I came across The **CONCUSSION LEGACY FOUNDATION**. While their focus is primarily athletes and military Veterans, and educating sports teams to be aware, and pro-active about protecting and detecting concussions, I began opening up all of their pages and links. Potential Dementia showing up all over the website.

Suddenly I did not feel so alone. So half-nuts. It added to my HOPE tool kit.   Further reading, I saw that they have a Brain Bank, dedicated to the study of multiple hits. In a half-laugh, I joked to myself, "Hey by golly, I think I qualify for something, at last!" Hoot! Hoot!

I contacted the foundation to learn about donating my brain upon my death. I kinda need it for a bit longer! I now have a message on my fridge and in my wallet, of my wishes to continue to serve, after my death, through science.

I asked permission to share about the Concussion Legacy Foundation, and the VA-BU-CLF Brain Bank. Upon submitting your email, they will send you wonderful information about their work. Even if you are not the recipient of multiple head injuries, I highly recommend that you visit the website at: www.concussionfoundation.org.

Once I started on this Google searching for info on my dad's condition, I saw Alzheimers and Dementia coming up over and over. Confused which was which, I found The Alzheimer's Association®. There, they gave great details of signs to look for, caregiver support, research advancements, and explained that Dementia is the umbrella term for many types of brain disease and conditions. Alzheimers being one.

I noticed that they hold several types of fundraiser and advocacy events throughout the year, with the biggest one being in the month of June, named: Alzheimer's & Brain Awareness month -   supporting the fight against this devastating disease. During the month, people all around the world are asked to wear purple in support. The Organization encourages folks to host and/or participate in an annual, global event called: The Longest Day. Ironically, that is my birthday. June 21st. The Summer Solstice. Something in my head said, if I can get this book done, and share what has happened to me and my dad, I will participate. At the time of this final edit, I plan to throw a birthday party, music jam and raise some funds, in memory of my dad, and... have some greatly-needed FUN! If this interests you to host your own event, I suggest you check out their very informative website. www.alz.org.

CHAPTER 4 - I Did Not Feel Alone

At some point after my Dr J. experience, I stumbled on to something wonderful. A TBI conference being held in Seattle. The idea of going to the city, traffic & travel - when I had barely driven a single highway to Bellingham, scared me. Mostly, because the first time I drove on our busy I-5, a 3-lane interstate, my head did a number. As cars passed, and the on-coming other lanes passed, I felt myself going backward. It terrified me. I wanted to stop in the middle of my lane and shrink. Hide under the seat or something. But managed to get off I-5 and recover. It took another month before I tried that again. And it was better. Good ol' TIME!

I contacted the Washington State TBI conference. I noticed on their website they were giving away scholarships for two nights stay by the airport where the conference was being held. Otherwise, it was around $300. I certainly could not afford that. So I applied and got an email a few days later, that I was accepted. May 2014. Wow! I was nervous.

May finally rolled around. I prayed a lot and took off to Seatac airport about 2 ½ hour drive south for me. I got lost at the airport and began to panic. But pulled over, took some deep breaths. Asked for help. I was so tired. I managed to find the hotel. Each little thing was so taxing. Parking. Checking in. Then carpet patterns. The smell of the chlorine pool. The fear of losing my cell phone, room and car key. Where to go in the A.M. to register. Times. Schedules and

PEOPLE. Lots and lots of people.

First thought was, OH MY GOSH, I want to go home. My farm. My doggies. My daughter. My miniature horses. My land. My house. My bed. My dirt. I had to do a lot of deep breathing. I saw people checking in, in all kinds of mental shapes. Wheelchairs, canes. dark glasses. Some with lil' therapy doggies. Most with a caregiver or spouse. And, me. Alone.

I have come to believe there are no mistakes when I boost up my faith, and know that everything is happening right on track. (I have listened to a lot of late, great, motivational author/speaker, Wayne Dyer.) When I remember this, the panic part lessens and the intrigue begins to grow.

I managed to get myself registered and, like cattle we all moved toward the big conference ballroom filled with round tables and a platform for the speaker. My balance gets wacky with many people walking, so I stayed near the wall.

I could not believe how many lights and again with the wild carpet patterns everywhere. It was a challenge to stay grounded and not fall over dizzy. But I was there. And the Washington State TBI Conference gave me the scholarship. So I was very grateful! And was gonna stick it out!

The keynote speaker began, welcomed us and we were off to 2 full days of learning about brain injury with wonderful resources available to us, little workshops, and some small talks with folks at my table. I even purchased a card with my injury information on it, that I carry in my wallet by my license.

By days-end I was wiped out. Ears ringing loudly. Headache thumpin. Ready for my room.

You had to buy your own supper so I went to the bar/restaurant with my little journal and all the literature they had provided. I could not believe what I had heard from survivors this first day. So much encouragement.

I reflected on one pinnacle moment that nearly made me choke on my lunch - when I looked up and around the room and saw myself in so many faces. **For the first time, in 6 long years, I did not feel alone.**

As I sat in the restaurant I noticed 4 men "checking me out" at a table next to me. I felt a little uncomfortable. The waiter returned for my order and asked if I wanted a drink. I had not drank anything for a long time. Why would I? Concussions make you feel drunk all the time! But he told me about a little famous local brew and I ordered the smallest scooner thinking it might calm my brain down.

The waiter asked me if I was there for the TBI conference and I said Yes. He smiled and walked away.   One of the fellas tossed me a question.   Something like "Where are you from?"   I told em. They said they were traveling salesmen from back east. Asking me what I was doing in Seattle, I told them briefly about my concussion stuff and that this was a big event, to learn more, and hopefully come away with hope.

They all seemed very interested. All said, "You would never know you had had a concussion. You are so twinkly and bright!" I smiled and nodded. I knew what my brain thought about that!

I ate my dinner. Jotted thoughts and was getting ready to head to my room, when 3 of the men got up and left. The 4th asked if he could sit with me a few minutes. Two thoughts came to mind: salesman gonna hit on girl, or he was going to ask about concussions. He sat down a few minutes. Asked about my concussion, in which I was very vague. "Oh just silly farm accident stuff". To shift the focus, I asked him about his life, family. Within a few minutes, I said I was tired and needed to go to my room.

I thanked the man for the little talk. Before I could stand up, he tapped my hand, and asked, "As you have been healing, I have to ask you something... have you been getting your needs met?" Shocked, I replied, "Excuse me?" He came back with: "You know, your *needs*?" I shook my head. It felt like a bad movie. A holy crap moment. It was everything for me not to switch to my Ellie Mae Clampet and grab the dude by the short hairs and toss him around the room! The nerve!

This guy was trying to score at a motel with a head-injured woman! I took a deep breath, released my tightening fist and I said, "You know, I am going to pretend I did not hear you ask that, and I am going to hope you go back to your room and call your wife and children. Goodnight!" Grrrrrr.

Really made me think about how vulnerable we can be. And how there are just low-life, lost souls, waiting to score on the wounded. Funny, if I would have seen this happening to another woman, I might have become a grizzly bear and he would have heard MUCH more. I tend to do that to protect others. Maybe even more now.

It was hard to sleep in the motel. For being fancy schmancy it was pretty noisy. The room smelled like cleaning products. The sheets smelled like bleach. The pillows were crunchy noisy. And I was far away from home. All new for me.

I managed to get to the breakfast the next morning. The florescent lights were painful on sleepy eyes and tired brain. But, I did get there in time to hear the keynote speaker. He was so funny and obvious that walking was difficult. It was hard to understand his words a bit too, but wow, really funny and inspiring. So honest about who he had been. He shared how his ego had been so big before his motorcycle accident. How he had to find the golden thread to keep going and how his life shifted to service. I was amazed.

A copy of his book was in our Survive and Thrive conference bags. An amazing man. I emailed him years later. He was very encouraging to me. He had had a stroke, since I heard him speak, and unable to walk or talk much, but still trying to figure out how to serve others through his journey. So inspiring.

Later, in the lobby, sitting by the fireplace sipping a cup of coffee, a woman sat down across from me. Lovely energy around her. Very calm. We got to talking. I told her a little as she asked about my journey. I even told her that after one injury, I produced 16 songs for a humanitarian project. How I barely remember actually producing or writing, but I did it. And, one song involved many people all saying the same message: WE ARE ONE. 19 languages from all over the world.

This woman told me she was astounded by my story. I asked if she was a survivor. I had never even used this language before. But that was the talk of the day. Survivor/thriver. THAT part - I liked a lot! The woman told me that she was a caregiver of her brain-injured son. Who was in very rough shape. Not the same young man. Bike accident without a helmet. I asked if he was attending. She said, no. Just her.

I realized the next speaker would be talking soon and wanted to get back. I thanked her for our time and headed back. They served up a nice lunch and then a voice stepped up to the podium. "I am the caregiver of my incredible son, who was not wearing a helmet and was in a bicycle accident. My life, his life, will never be the same." Turns out my lovely talk by the fireplace was the keynote speaker. Wow. I purchased her book afterward that was full of small steps in recovery and contact information for the "system" out there, when life changes radically.

A gentleman stepped up after her talk was over and told about his brain injury that had happened 30 years prior. I could not believe how people were still battling the symptoms. It actually scared me. I needed a little break from the weird lights and went out in the hall to get a cup of coffee. When I turned around, I saw a tall, slender man standing in the doorway of the conference listening to the speaker. Get this! He had a very long pony tail! Could it be? Hmmmm.

A little twinge of "Irish moxy" went through me and I walked straight up behind him and said, "Hello, Dr. J." He turned around and stepped back in surprise and said a surprised hello. Appearing a bit shocked, he said, "I have spoken at this before and was on my way back from Tacoma and thought I would stop in."

I did not smile or frown. Straight-faced, I said, "It took everything I had to get to this, and unlike my appointment with you, here, this conference is giving me hope." Then I pointed to the man speaking and asked, "Do you know why I have hope? See that man up there? He is a survivor. He knows my journey from the inside out. He understands." Then, I looked at him with no emotion and said, "Goodbye" and walked back in the conference room.

Now please understand something - I am not like this. I am gentle, listening, a spiritual heart that learns from everything and everyone. (Unless you intend harm to my loved-ones, then well, I am a little bear cat!)

Dr. J taught me something huge in this foggy journey. He represented the professional intellect that can tell us what pill we can try. Can matter-of-fact document dates, and assess our motor and cognitive abilities... but, they cannot actually identify, unless, they are the rare soul that perhaps had a parent with mental illness, or loved-one who had a stroke or concussion. They are an outsider looking in at facts. The horrible part is, even with MRIs they cannot see all the damage. Nor do they have any idea how long it will take to heal or if you ever will.

See, that is the kicker here. I do not poo poo going to a neurologist. I also do not poo poo counselors - but here again, I caution who you see. The next chapter will explain why.

Chapter 5 - 10 Damn More Minutes!

Through the years, just about the time I would get to thinkin' that maybe the new fog was deciding to stay, like, *forever...* something amazing would happen.

Summer of 2016, I was back in action with my farming. Growing food to donate to the food banks and feeling good. I ended up writing a song, from my tractor, called: **Who will feed the hungry**. I made a homegrown music video for you tube and was suddenly in the news advocating, my farm's mantra: "grow and give", to feed our hungry. It felt great. September came and I found myself coordinating a food drive, with the help of Bellingham's Unity church and, shining a light on Washington's *Northwest Harvest*. I even went to Seattle to meet the staff that provides nearly 2 million meals a month and have been feeding Washington's hungry for over 50 years. I was blown away by the amazing volunteers. I should add here, that the following year I got a call from Country Woman Magazine, who heard about my efforts, loved my grow to give story and published it the follow fall to 300,000 readers. Amazing blessings!

While I did not smack my head again, with all the busyness, I was not sleeping well. The stress of pulling this calling together was almost too much. But I was lit up and wanted to help others.

My family doc suggested I see a counselor when I told her I was not feeling stable. Some days good. Some days all the sudden incredibly dark and low. The doc's office called with a name of a counselor that had TBI experience. Yay! This felt hopeful and pro-active for me. Unfortunately, I had to cancel the first attempt at an appointment due to a 5-day migraine. So - we reschedule. The food drive came and went, and in 3 hours we gathered enough food to feed about 1500 people. It was worth the stress.

The day of my new appointment, with my finances running very low, I had someone coming to buy a travel trailer, which would give me some cash. This single-mom, low-income stuff was stressful enough. The timing was bad. The buyer was traveling from 3 hours away and was running late. My appointment was at 1. I do not do well with this type of stuff.

I could see I was going to be 10 - 15 minutes late if I drove like a crazy woman, 25 minutes to town. I called the counselor's office and told her I may be late. She quickly replied, "Well, Laurie, you will be billed anyway, so get here!"

I drove fast, plus had a big headache. I arrived only about 5 minutes late. Found parking and ran (NOT suppose to jar my brain by running) found her address, flew up the steep flight of steps, and went to where she said to wait in a waiting room. Down the hall, I could see a woman on a phone. I waved and smiled. No response. She looked straight at me and kept talking. I glanced at the clock on the wall. Said 1:10. Just then, she shut the door. What? At 1:20 the woman came out, gestured me down the hall. I hustled and apologized.

Trust me, this is going somewhere!

I got right in and got to business. Thanked her and perhaps was speaking fast. Adrenaline. I laid out that I wasn't really sure where to start with healing but feeling the blues lately even during a wonderful humanitarian project (that was on the front cover of the newspaper) I wanted to talk about depression and healing.

I showed her my many head bonks on a little paper that I brought with me, knowing she knew all about TBI. No, I did not bring Thumper, the styrofoam head. She was sleeping!

I told her about my divorce, moving many times through my life, some abuse stuff, care-giving my parents at the other end of the farm and, the many bonks. But how good stuff had come from it too. Producing CDs, farming, and a deeper spiritual sense to life. She did not say much. Took notes. Did not look at me. Then at one point she finally looked up and asked me, "Why don't you just move off of your farm so you will stop hitting your head?" I chuckled with surprise. I said, "The farm has been my medicine. Even if I have hit some on the farm, others were flukes away from my home."

The counselor insisted that moving would be best. I was getting a little frustrated. I told her that was not an option at the time to just walk away, and that my elderly parents live on the other end of the farm in rough shape. Then I asked her, "Have you ever played in the dirt? Cut gorgeous bouquets from flowers you have grown, or gathered your harvest of food from your own soil? That is medicine!" Her reply over her reading glasses was: "I will ask the questions!"

At one point, I remember her dog-legging off on to something she did in her own life. Honestly, I felt the clock ticking. It seemed wrong and unfair to me!

The clock said 1:50. I thought, okay, maybe the last 10 minutes, we would get down to business or we will go over, seeins' how she was 10 minutes late too. My head was starting to really pound and felt very tired from all that yappin' my life story and the rush to get there. Suddenly, the counselor stood up with the chart board in her hand, glanced at her notes and then again over her reading glasses said, "Laurie, I do not think I can help you. Most of my clients come in with some idea of what they want to work on. You have many things."

I was stunned. Absolutely stunned. I asked, "Isn't it your job to help someone find a starting place when they show up to do the work, to try to heal?" Her reply, "Yes, Laurie, but I just don't think I can help you." well, alrighty then. All this, and *I had 10 damn more minutes!*

I could not believe the day. The rush and danger to get there. The stress. The headache. Running! And, she could not help me. I stood up and squared off with her and said, "Okay, well, this was interesting. When I arrived, you saw me, did not smile, made me wait 10 minutes, closed your door on me, so you could finish a phone call on *my time*. We spoke when you were finally ready. I tried very hard to share. Now, you have closed the door on me again saying you cannot help me, because I don't have a starting point. Wow and um, Wow!"

She stumbled on her next few words, adjusting her glasses, and said with a slight chuckle, "Well, if you would like to set up another appointment, perhaps we could try this again." My reply, "Or, perhaps not. Thanks. Adios!" Grrr.

I share this experience again, not because this is the normal counselor experience - but it *is* my intention to share so *IF* you get a crappy neurologist or counselor or any doctor - maybe my story will help somehow. You or your loved-one are entitled to respect, first and foremost. You went through the hell. Because you went through that hell, they make a living! They would not have a job if we never got messed up and took the time to go to them. Now and then, THEY need to be reminded!

If anything, I 'spose all of this is making me have to stand up for myself. But dang it has been exhausting! I think I ended up taking a Gabapentin when I got home because my brain started zapping. That has been one medicine I keep available. When my brain gets flying out of control in 10 directions... it seems to reset the noodle somehow. I know it doesn't work for everyone. So I feel fortunate.

I also went back to my herb/vitamin books and researched again for help and found B-COMPLEX is critical when depression comes. Ginko Biloba really does help with several areas of my brain. Recall, blues, headaches. If I stay on it. Magnesium to relax muscles and sleep. Which in my case, after trying Melatonin, Zquill, Tylonel PM, I recently switched to the lowest dose of Trazadone. Sleep deprivation is brutal. The brain cannot heal without it. I realized the vicious circle and have finally agreed to take something to conk out for a couple nights. I am still working on this part! Again, one KEY healing ingredient is: SLEEP!

My family doc wanted me to try Amitriptiline, which helped with sleep for a few nights, and then, back-fired like I had drank a bunch of coffee. You get tired of trying pills. Herbs. Vitamins. Research. But don't give up. Keep trying.

One thing I will say- I discovered that is really good for anxiety... and may replace my Gabapentin seizure med is 5-HTP aka Triptiphan. The stuff in turkey that makes you fall asleep after Thanksgiving dinner while burping with a big ol' belly - from eating too much.

To close this chapter, I just want to remind you, that if you or a loved one hits your head, one of the most critical things we can do, is take note. Tell someone. Remember. Write it down. And watch. My TBI/concussions following the first and biggest in 2008, had a pattern. First WHOP. Ouch. Within minutes, my left side of my face primarily my jaw, lips and left nostril would go numb.   And stay anywhere from a day to 3.   But the balance, headaches, dizzy spells, motor skills, speech, eye swelling pressure - all would arrive about day 3! Which, I have learned, symptoms can slowly creep in even up to two weeks later!   THIS IS IMPORTANT STUFF. STUFF I never knew could be possible.

Well, by now, you might be wanting to ask *"HOW THE*

HECK DID YOU HIT YOUR HEAD SO MANY TIMES AND WHAT DID YOU HIT IT ON?" Even I laugh and shake my head at this part. I will share *all* of them bonkies in Chapter 8. Thumper's List. Kinda makes me blush with embarrassment still in telling how these goofy things can happen.

But first, I have a few more thangies to say!

No idea why these poems want to come out. I just touch the keys and boom. Written.

Hurry up, hurry up, door is closing!
Late for this appointment of mine -
So sorry, so sorry, I drove like hell!
Doc, I'm waiting on you - this time.

Waiting room, weird perfume,
the clock says 15 minutes late!
Tell me your story, quickly Laurie,
And I'll schedule another date.

What the heck, who is the doc?
You just told me your life woes-
that'll be - $130 please,
Pay up doc, cuz I gotta go!
LLL

Chapter 6 - Mo Betta!

About 4 years after Dr. J, another thump put me back in the neurological black hole again. I heard about a new doctor, who was taking patients. Young and really just setting up his practice.

I was hesitant, but also on a desperate page to talk. My Thumper styrofoam head was getting more flags with dates of hits. Honestly, I felt a little bonkers.

I arrived and met the doc. Quiet, kind, gentle. He was very curious about my condition. Not in disbelief. Not poo pooing that I was not an athlete that got clobbered by a 300 pound defense, he just listened. It took a bit for him to read me. Partly because I am sparkly sometimes. So someone seeing me, with my makeup on, hair brushed, it is a lil' hard to compute. He did the typical tests for tracking and balance. And offered some sleep suggestions. I did not let him meet Thumper - the first appointment.

He suggested I take Gabapentin, but a lower dose more often to keep my mind from multi-tracking and zinging out of control. So I did this for awhile and it helped. This doctor was a MO BETTA blessing, that I seriously needed after Dr. T. and Dr. J.

He was also a musician and it was nice to see his expression when I said I had lost my music abilities for 6 months - from one of the hits. Gone. Poof. It helped us connect at how we take life for granted. Of we assume our thoughts and abilities we have today, will be there tomorrow. But thump, maybe not.

Over the course of the next few years, I had a couple appointments with him and he met Thumper. He was also more than willing to help me with disability papers if I went that route. He was also very encouraging and impressed at what I have done with my life - even with injuries.

So even though Dr. J was a bad experience, in a way it wasn't. Because, I am writing about it. Warning YOU. And isn't that pretty dang cool? Guess I am a guinea pig or lab rat of life. Luckily the tests have not killed me yet.

So try to keep all of this in mind (loaded words) when you begin the search for a brainyologist.... they are not all the same.

In May of 2018, my daughter drove me to a brain specialist in Seattle who also was in almost disbelief that a simple farm gal could hit her head so many times. While our appointment did not start out very good, and honestly, I felt her intelligence filling the room rather that any compassion, until, I said, "I DID NOT COME HERE FOR DISABILITY, I came here for HOPE." Then added, "May you never hit your head doc, and be unable to open the computer, drive to work, type, fight depression, think, walk, talk... and then, try to explain your horror - to doctor like you."

It was in these words that tears of pure intention and honesty broke loose, looking at her in that shitty, over-lit florescent exam room. She shifted. She actually shifted. When I told her I was writing a book, she said, "I would like to read your book. I believe you."

Heavy clouds,

pouring rain -

brought mega fog

to my brain -

but I persisted,

to buck through the weatha -

found a new doc,

Now feel - mo betta!

Cheesy lil' poem but true!

Thanks Dr... (Shhhh)

Please keep caring.

LLL

Chapter 7 - Thumper and Words

Before I share my thumps and bumps, WORDS and their importance popped into my head. So I guess that needs to be shared first.

Remember in the movie Bambi, Thumper's mama asked, "Thumper, what did your father say?" Lil Thumper bunny touches his ears and with a big sigh and adorable little voice says, *"If you can't say nothin' good, don't say nothin' at all."*

I love that.   I *really* love that.   I joke about my nickname as Thumper. At first it was out of embarrassment, I think. But now, when I call myself or my styrofoam head *Thumper* - I think rather than put myself down for hitting my noggin' so many times - I lift myself up to say: "BRAVO, LAURIE, you have been down the rabbit hole or black hole of hell in your life, not just concussions (but that's another story) but you have worked so hard to come back up.

There were times on this journey when others have had some pretty insensitive opinions. Like accusing me of faking it so I did not have to get a job. Meanwhile, I could not drive or barely walk down the hall without bashing into the walls." Or this one that hurt when I was told by someone: "My sister has seizures and she is fine."   Or this ouchie: "You are not a good caregiver to your father and mother."

Talk about head injury... my dad was post-stroke. That is a doozy! Or the lovely comments like: "You hit your head again? What, do you have, like a death wish, or trying to knock some sense into yourself?" Or how 'bout this one which I will not say how many have said this one to me (all because they cared) "YOU NEED TO WEAR A HELMET 24/7, Laurie" and while I know they mean well, I really don't have an interest in wearing a helmet that creates the same pressure I already have dealt with for years. I tried it. Threw the sucker across the room!

Or maybe this one, that still makes me laugh, after a neighbor once asked, "Where have you been, Laurie? Have not seen you out on the farm." I softly and quickly answer, "I bumped again" and before I could finish the word "again", I hear: "Oh my God, I don't even want to hear about it. Too stressful!" Ya think!

Words are so powerful. I saw it with my mom trying to deal with my dad's post-stroke brain, that ended with Dementia. It killed me to know how horrible it was for her *and* him. He became a different man. I tried to remind her that he was trying his best. Anger makes anger. To somehow try to emphasize the good. Try to make the last chapter and the inevitable the best they could. But I understand too well, how horrible it can be. It was.

I know for many of us, too much information at once makes the mind swirl. Many people talk without checking in with you, to see if you are still tracking. I have a paranoia about talking too much. I am sure I do when I am on a roll. There were many months where I barely talked at all. Not at ALL on the telephone. I couldn't. Made my head feel like it was going to burst. And partially because my sentences came out scrambled. Sometimes my daughter would look at me and say "Huh?"   I searched for words. Or when I would try to talk, I would end up with someone who was pretty dang sure they knew what you were going to say – if stalling or stuttering, searching for words, so they'd either steal the sentence or finish it. Sure glad when that fog lifted!

Then there are those that rattle on forever with every

gnats-ass, finite detail of where, when, first/last name of the person in the story, color of the sky, etc... and you just wanted to scream GET TO THE PUNCH LINE PLEASE! But we don't. We are polite. We might be swirling inside. Wanting them to, um, honestly.... shut up!

One I am still not sure how to adjust to, is the one when an evening or talk is going along beautifully and positively, when suddenly the subject of politics and the state of our country come out. The energy in the person I am talking with suddenly shifts to the BIG, strong, opinion – filled with anger and blame and despair. I have been known to come back with my wee portion of good juju to say, FEAR CANNOT WIN if we don't let it.   Of course I am sure I sound like a looney to one that chooses to be so up on the news. It is so draining.

I know all this sounds unkind, but when you are duct-taped together, trying to survive not just a day, but an hour, a few minutes... you can get pretty over-whelmed. I felt so bad for my daughter and her dad when the fog was really thick.

Words.   This was a problem and probably killed my marriage. Aside from me clinging to spiritual faith for hope, and he had become atheist and could not understand why faith was important -   I was   also married to a lovely, very intelligent, scientific man. I admired his brain, but needed simplicity during the fog - not over explanations. Tiny little things became such long talks.   Many options and ways suggested to do just about anything. Words, words, words. Remember I said in the beginning of the book, that as a songwriter, I get 3 ½ minutes or so - to tell you what I need to say? BINGO!

I will say, my ex-husband was amazing during the hell. He knew so much about my condition. He saw some ugly, sad stuff. Coming home from work to find his dazed and confused/sad wife still wearing the same shirt, inside out. Un-brushed hair. Far away look in my eyes. Dishes stacked up. No dinner. Maybe weeping. (Man, this is hard to write.) We developed words that did cut me some slack. They were these: "Good day? Bad day?" Each day when he would come home, he would ask. At first, day after day, it was: bad day. Then a good day would appear and the thick fog would start to lift. Slowly more good days returned. Thank you, Wes.

Both my daughter and her daddy knew there were triggers that would flip my head out. Camera flashes, Fluorescent lights, loud bass music, gun shots, fragrances, carpet smells, diesel fumes, busy motion in movies, carnivals, too many people talking, even traffic... all of it was so hard for me and them. I was no fun at all! My daughter knew never to wave her hands in front of my eyes for it could set off a seizure. NOT FUN! Certainly not the life of the party!

Well I guess I am stalling on the actual THUMPER'S LIST of bonks. I reckon that is the Chapter that wants to be written next ... but I really wanted to drive home how important it is to create positive words, keep things simple, otherwise, holy crap it becomes: TMI to a TBI can lead to TMJ and PIA, aka pain in ass! LOL. Isn't it funny how 3 letters are the new language!

One more very important thing about words. I know a few, that, while sugar is not good for the brain, these words are like candy. Dad taught me this. When the brain is struggling, be it concussion or Dementia, we don't feel very smart. So when a loving heart says sugar words like this, it is fabulous medicine or at least calming: "GOOD JOB! You are RIGHT about that! That's right! I forgot!" Lol! Anything to make another person feel good instead of, frankly... dumb!

Words are powerful! What we say. So is: *listening*. We have become a society of piss-poor listeners. So eager with opinion. Or not listening at all. Distracted by our techy toys, phones, a book or TV or computer... So it isn't always what we say, it can be: do we listen?

I had a friend tell me once, "You are a very good listener Laurie, and you try harder than anyone I know, to remember what is said." That was so nice to hear. Thank you, Bob.

Because I forgot as soon as I would say something, often, trying to hold my thought when a long-winded person would steal my sentence just to hear themselves yap - it was so difficult. Again wanting to just burst out with WHERE ARE OUR MANNERS and COMMON CURTIOUSY?!

I loved how someone I felt close to would say something to me two or three times. Repeat stories. And not remember that they had told me at the last very rare restaurant luncheon. Where I would struggle to listen. Retain. And honestly, treasure our visit. I would laugh inside when maybe a month later, see them again and hear the same story. Realizing, hells bells, you can have concussions, and believe it or not, make conversations MORE memorable or valuable than those with no troubles at all... because you know NEVER to take memory or conversations for granted. You might not get another chance! Make it count!

Okay... this might take a bit... we are going to travel back to July 2008 when all was well in Laurie's world. Yup yup yup!

Remember, this is being written by the chick who has survived and thrived... after a whole lotta thumpin' was goin' on! Sounds kinda kinky. Uh, not! Next Chapter, how you hit yer head many times in 10 years.

You could try to make all of this stuff up... but I am just NOT that creative!

Chapter 8 – Thumper's list

"She with most hits does not win ... or does she?"

1. The beginning. Back of my head. July 2008, while simply shampooing an area rug, bent down to adjust shampooer and came up full speed under 40 lb steel hanging lamp and fell to the ground. Symptoms unfolded in the next 2 weeks. Saw 2 docs. Slurred speech. Tipping over, headaches, swollen eyes. Stuttered. No driving.

2. Feeling a bit better. Oct 2008. walked into our lower barn, to check on the goats, bent, came up and smacked right into a 2 x 6 " low hanging beam. Almost the same spot as bonk 1. Instant dizzy. Off balance. Face began to tingle. Could barely make it to the house. All the symptoms returned. So many headaches. Walked like a duck. Motor skills off.

3. Still not well, Nov. 2008, went to Seattle for then husband's birthday party. Rented house with family with low ceilings ... night was going good until bed. Heading up stairs, turned to say goodnight. I hit hard on the low stair landing. Instant goose egg front right of forehead. Shook. Afraid to go to sleep. Laid awake by daughter all night. Symptoms back.

4. I got 2009 off. It was incredible. Celebrated. Made it to July 2010! Was singing with family at a concert outdoor. Finished. I remembered all the words. Was so happy. Putting equipment in back of our truck, hubby slammed canopy door down on the front side of my head. Instant rattle. Numb face. Symptoms followed. So many headaches.

BIG FOG: Sept. 2010 had to have full blown hysterectomy. Everything changed. Sudden menopause at 47 and severe healing window. This was horrible. More fog. So much pain. And now, hot flashes, chills, highs and lows. Migraines.

5. March 2011 had big headache and stopped at my folks. Construction was happening. 2 x 12 beam blocked door. I bent under it to go under and came up to fast, pow. Big hit in the back of my head. By the time I got inside face was numb. Headache. And slurred speech. Seizure (triple vision began) for a 6-month window.

6. June 2011, working on chicken barn, wearin a baseball cap, the brim blocked my view and I came up under a chunk of plywood. Damn it! Saw stars!

7. July 2011 - Still feeling the last hit, went to pump gas to take friend and go stay at a lovely retreat house for a night. Pumping gas, wind came up and wham! Door slammed and caught the side of my head. How my head gets in these places is beyond me. By the time I drove, I knew I was in rough shape. Went anyway. Not so fun!

8. Finally a break of 9 months. Then Sept 2011 Then hit hard on a shelf in our school room. Symptoms came in about 3 days. Balance, headaches, dizzy, walking funny.

9. YAY, no hits again for almost a year... then June 2012, saddling a horse, going to try to take a family ride. Bent down to get the cinch and stirrup fell. Boom. By the time we got to the place to ride I was already feeling swirled. Dazed. Numb face. Not tracking well.

10. June 2012 Just 2 days after stirrup thump, had to go get hay for winter. Just told a gal was on a roll. Only hit once couple days ago. Wasn't feeling good but got hay anyway. No more than said I am done hitting and I tipped head back fast and smacked steel bar in our truck. Dang!

11. Aug. 2012 just a couple months later, feeling a bit better, was out fixing fence with horses. Old busy head POCO horse came up to help. I bent to pic up pliers and when coming up, our heads collided. I said

ouch. Poco was fine. Omgosh. This was horrible. I cried.

12. Mar 2013. wearing cowboy hat, went in chicken barn. As I do, daily. Hit beam coming out. Jeez . Numb face, wacky balance and so on.

13. June 2013 Still not 100% trying to rush to make a nice dinner for family, went in bathroom. Bent over and smacked towel bar hard. Came up and everything was spinning.

14. July 2013, just a month later, bathing our dog, stood up fast and fell backward into a big cedar pole of our deck. Smack. Ring. Face went numb. Spent that night alone. Scared. Felt very nervous.

15. March 2014. Down trying to work on little pony barn, turned, lost balance and fell into the side of the building, slamming my head. Could barely get to the house.

16. May 2014 trying to do yard work, with weed eater... I hit a big branch of pear tree. Damn. Cut that sucker off!

17. June 2014 -This was not a hit. This was a jarring. This was horrible. Went with a friend in a farm truck to deliver raspberries about 30 miles south. The seat I was in had a big spring and bounced hard the whole trip. And back. When I came home my eyes swelled huge and for next 2 weeks, hell. As like the other hits

18. July 2014 Sitting in a lawn chair, leaned back and fell backward and hit the corner of the patio door. Everyone heard this.

19. BIG ugly hit. Made it to Nov 2014. Had my truck parked under patio roof. Loading stuff to move a friend. Stepped up in bed of truck full speed and hit a 2 x 6 beam. Dropped me to my knees. Continued to move friend and realized I had no idea I was driving. Big symptoms followed.

20. Un-stinkin believable... August 2015.. simply got out to open my farm gate. Wind blowing so hard could barely push it. Opened door of Explorer, got in and wind blew door wham against my head.

ENOUGH ALREADY!

And then ...*enough already*... happened! Yup Yup. I had a 2-year break. Two glorious years. I needed all my faculties because my mom and dad both had big medical needs. But then...

21. August 2017, luck ran out...

Leaning into my Ford Ranger truck to get something I clobbered my forehead on the steel frame. Saw stars. That one only gave me symptoms for a couple weeks. YAY. Numb face being one of them. Always freaky, wondering if you are actually having a stroke!

22. June 2018, Wacko. This one is embarrassing, Simply reaching into my fridge, it is low, lost balance, and hit the latch that closes the fridge, came out fast and hit the back of my head on the bottom of the freezer portion. Woohoo. Two spots in one goofy action of getting cream cheese. Two bruises.

23. August 2nd, 2018. My dad dying in the nursing home. The morning before he died. All I did was go out and saw choke weed taking over my fence and little plants. Started pulling. Harder and harder, thinking of my dad's miserable last 24 days and me having to do it all. I yanked the hell out of that vine and BAM. Sent backward like a fist came through the bushes. I pulled a pole down that had a screw sticking out. It hit the left part of my forehead. Immediate goose-egg and blood and a big bruise. Best part, I had so much grief and stress going on, I don't even remember the symptoms. At least this one swelled out, rather than in.

It seems like most of the wacky symptoms of each of hit arrived about day 3. The worst of the symptoms like not tracking, balance, migraines, swollen eyes, agitated, depressed, seizure-type episodes, tipping over, unable to drive, or do math, or write in cursive walk like a duck were all pretty scary. Some would happen immediately. The numb face. Sometimes hard to swallow. Unsure if I had food in my mouth, stuff like that. Symptoms would last anywhere from 2- 3 weeks, to the big hits. 3-4 months. Whew!

But even with all these hits... life went on. I still farmed and I tried to do family functions. When the fog would lift, I was be so eager to get going again. Quick to forget those massive headaches and symptoms. Happy to be alive.

As I said, some incredible things happened in between hits. This head injury stuff can bounce you from the foggy surreal what is going on, to the deepest darkest scary pits of how will I survive today, this hour, the next minutes... without faith and hope of a better tomorrow, there were times I admit a bullet in that noggin to remove the unbelievable pain and fog seemed like it would have been better.

As I write this, and journey back through, and see how many incredible people I have met, songs I have written, charities I have helped, and how much love I have experienced... I would not change a thing. Shoot, this was only a 10-year window... all the years before took me pretty close to the edge too. Apparently this head-bonking decade really wanted to teach me about self-worth, learning to become more and more present and grateful NOW.

All the King's horses and all the King's men...
could not put Laurie's head back together again.

MEDICINE: TIME, HOPE and FAITH.

Kinda freaky, aint it? Impossible? A singing farm chick. Not even an athlete!

Sadly, one concussion alone kinda shows its best healing progress in about a year. When ya whop and whop they kinda tie themselves together.

When you are heading into the washing machine MRI

tube for the 4ᵗʰ time, and the Xray tech reads multiple concussions... you know they must be wondering "Who the heck is this girl?" The only good thing I got from those dag gum noisy MRIs was the fact that it proved I was NOT a hypochondriac! They did have to tell me not to move several times, when I was listening to Elvis on the headphones! But hey, it was scary and he was "Blue Suede Shoeing" to me!

Without faith and hope of a better tomorrow, there were times I admit a bullet in this noggin to remove the unbelievable pain and fog seemed like it would have been better. But as I write this, and journey back through, and see how many incredible people I have met, songs I have written, charities I have helped, and how much love I have experienced, I would not change a thing.

This head-bonking chapter really wanted to teach me about self-worth and learning to become more and more present to NOW and gratitude.

Writing this book, I am amazed how many emotions have surfaced. I have finished paragraphs laughing, crying, angry, sad, shaking, and grateful.

Wait til I share about what it is like to have a dented head and broken heart and then - try to love again.

Are you still with me? Its quite a story, huh? Yah, I am still alive typing this, woohoo! Amazed myself actually. That's us folks! We are made of unbelievable stuff!

My story is no more dramatic than yours.

I just have had a lot of things happen in chunks of time. Most the time, this stuff can be turned into gold of inspiration and connectedness, if we are willing to honor the fog, learn from it, and share what we learned when it lifts!

Ya know, I mentioned anger just above here. I talk a lot about how the emotions get all screwed up. I consider myself very fortunate over this long haul, to not be full of rage and anger during the times the fog has been the thickest. It would be easy to stay in that place when symptoms could last not days - but weeks, even months.

Don't get me wrong, I HAVE gotten pissed off. I HAVE said F it, when family started adding salt to the wounds. I have told off some of the boards and beams that clobbered my head! I aint no angel. Or if I am, hehe, I have a few black feathers in my wings.

In the next chapter, I do have some stuff to share about anger, that probably could help anybody. Mom use to call it the "shit fits" of dad's personality... hmm. So it makes you wonder: if you start out shitty fittier... what happens when your brain is altered?

Since that whole symptom stuff was pretty heavy and we are now going to talk some about anger, thought I would end on a lighter tone. Be prepared though, it is quite profound. Quite deep and meaningful. Quite, um, well, you will see.

To end this chapter and set you up for the next. The best visual came to me about this idea of anger and spewing or blaming someone else for your misery who is in ear-shot. It goes something like this:

I remember hearing an old man say to a neighbor's big ol' black lab... that crossed the road specifically to crap in the old man's yard:

"Damn you dog, this is my yard and I don't want your shit, so keep it in your butt and GO HOME!"

BAHAHAHAHA!
Gotcha!

Please take a moment here in silence, ponder
this wisdom, and visualize the above story!
Tis good therapy!

Did I mention how good humor is, for healing?
Laughter is organic medicine.
Unless of course, like me, you have a weak bladder!

Chapter 9 - Anger and Volcanoes

I want to confess or address an ouch here. You are my confession booth. I am not Catholic so I have never really experienced confession. Something that has haunted my heart for a long time regarding anger. Maybe, if I share it, I can release it.

Pretty weird writing a book like this - that exposes a soul so vulnerably. Hells bells, I might have to look at the "look" others give me, for the rest of my life, since deciding to share my journey. But ya know what, that's okay. In a blink it can happen to anyone. And is. In another blink, I might not be here, but my experiences will. And if it helps another aka HOPE, awesome!

I have heard many stories about anger. I have seen it. You hear it a lot with Dementia. Where couples that have been married for 60 years, suddenly and so sadly, have to be separated because Grampa tried to kill Gramma. In a different head. My dad's Dementia did not get that far, but his post and pre-stroke were filled with anger. Short fused. More swear words than regular words. My mom was fit to be tied. I wondered how she held it together?

She didn't. She got a massive ulcer that combine with stress from care-giving my dad and having to take anti-inflammatory and pain medications for years for severe Osteoarthritis. Her ulcer blew and she almost bled to death. Guess who saved her? My dad. I get a call at 4 A.M. By a shaky lil guy sayin, "Sis, ma is awful sick. Can you come here?

Not sure she is breathing." Oh my Gosh! I was there in minutes, because I am just 3 acres away. Dad was clear and able to save his wife. I praised him over and over in his fear of how GOOD he did. Lil guy, shuffling like Carol Burnett's Tim Conway, eyes big, trying to clean up the mess. Mom was in horrible shape when we got her to ER.

But when anger comes, it is hard to go through it. With some Dementia, anger can arrive quite often. Caregivers have to learn not to take it personally or they will lose it. Trust me, words typed here are just words typed here... til you go through this. Trying to change the focus and keep things simple to keep down the aggression. Any brain trauma can bring forth anger. As they teach caregivers: You must enter their world. Gentle, leaning and softening energy, touch, words are helpful. My brain does not do well with aggression. Anytime confrontation, blood pressure going up, adrenaline, etc... it makes my brain want to zap. So this was a tricky road with dad. And trying to get my family to give a damn.

In reality, you aren't actually the one they want to be angry at. But you are there. They are trapped in a vicious, thick fog. Again, this may be you, the one in the fog, reading this. We/they don't always have that clarity to even express that part or the awareness. Just surviving one moment at a time. The angry one may feel safe enough with this is extremely off-balance condition to let it out. It sure doesn't make sense to couples that have stayed married through thick and thin, for it to get so damn thick, and often scary at the end! Someone is left drained, confused, maybe even angry themselves of how much they gave, and then, that person died.

Mom's safety was constantly being monitored and life was changing. Dad had had several concussions 2 years before his stroke. It was down hill from there. Here I was, in rough shape too. Keeping up with two little people and my own life, trust me, this book is still a miracle to me!

So the one story I have, my confession, that bothers my conscience, to some, might seem trivial. My intention to write this was not to tell you what to do. It was what I went through. Then you take what you need if it can help you. Inside the injured brain, you are trapped. No matter how hard you try to fight your way out, as I keep saying, TIME and trying to become aware - is all you have.

In one of the fogs, we had several kitties. Tinkerbell, an old kitty, was wonderful. But then, she shifted where she would not eat. If she ate, she tossed it up. When you aren't tracking very well, it doesn't take much to effect the nerves. Seeing her suffer was terrible. Stepping in cat urp wasn't very nice either!

We finally took her to the vet. She had a tooth that needed to be extracted. She would meow so often through the day. A totally different cat. And, I was a different mom. We got the tooth fixed, she healed and began to eat again. Then a couple months later, it happened all over again. I did everything I could to make foods for her. It was draining to me.

My daughter and her dad kinda expected me to know what to do, or take care of her. It was on one of the days, (tummy tightener here) that she had cried and cried for food. I tried all kinds of food and my own day was going so badly with a migraine, to bend over to feed her, with a pounder plus bending made me feel like I was falling.

I was also trying to create a dinner. Which was a big mother to achieve when in the fog. Suddenly, the constant crying in the kitchen got me. I push-kicked Tinkerbell sending her across the kitchen floor. Not really hard but basically saying shut up! I have had enough. My ex came around the corner and reprimanded me for being mean. Oh my gosh, I broke to a gallon of tears and ran to the bedroom hollerin' back that I was the only one who gave a damn about trying to help that cat! Their turn!

Now, you might be reading this and say, "Really Laurie, that's it?" It's not it. I don't lose my temper, if I can help it. I try to re-channel it elsewhere. After having seizure episodes I have tried to really avoid conflict and ramped-up energy if I can. But of course you don't end up in divorce most the time without conflict/arguments - at least once. Sadly, I blew up at my dad once for his anger to my mom. Weird as that sounds, it stopped him, but did not help me. I had to take seizure medicine after the blow and walk/cry for an hour out in the field.

Anger lets you know a perspective of just how hard you are trying. Or if you have become so dependent on another so you blame them for your unhappiness. Your pain. For me, often thinking it WAS me, my limited thinking and such, I have had a hard time truly knowing when to tell someone to go to hell and back off, or walk away and feel like a shhhhmuck myself, for not standing up or mis-reading what was going on. Good ol' fear.

Part of this comes from an experience that stuck to my cells pretty deeply. In my late 20's I got myself into an abusive relationship that basically took one weekend to get into, and 2 years to get back out, alive. Yes, there was a window, where I saw what anger *out-of-control* can do. If you happen to be a gentle soul, you might get sucked in thinking love will help but sadly, it might get you almost killed. You might just be all alone with that out-of-control angry person, behind closed doors, being picked up by your neck and told, "if I can't have you, no one can." THAT is a scary wake-up call about our self-worth or how much is too much. A VERY thick fog! To this day, I owe a beautiful sister-soul a huge *thank you* for rescuing me from a fist swinging, screaming, crazy man in a truck! I would not be writing this book, had she not saved me. Thank you so much, Heidi.

We all get angry. It is there for a reason. Anger can be what gives someone the greatest courage to do the hardest things.   It is what we do with it or spew on someone that is the challenge. With brain injuries, drugged brains, stroke and Dementia brains... they are not operating at full capacity. Counseling might be very important, or intervention. Even medication. After all, the one who loves and stands by you – did not do this to you. It is not their fault. Blame and anger tend to hold hands.

Pretty important to read and remember. It is easy to want to blame someone.   Heck, I would smash my thumb, hit my shin, smack my elbows and I really REALLY wanted to scream at someone. But in reality, it was me. Grateful no one walked up about the time I did it. I have learned to breathe out through my oweee pain, like birthing – to get through some of some might big thumps. Not just my head. Horse kicked me in the knee, sent me flying. A refrigerator fell on top of me, flattened me and almost busted my knee cap. Fell through ladder and shin swelled huge. On and on.   I was glad I was alone to not be unkind to another. After all, I DID it! But if you do blow, for goodness sakes SAY YOU ARE SORRY!

I try to own my injuries, best I can.   Which can be pretty hard to do when you were just doing a simple farm or life task and whammo.

Hatred and anger can become pure poison to the soul. So no matter how hard we struggle to heal and lift our fog, that cloud isn't going to lift all the way.   Anger will hold it down and hover over our lives.   I speak from personal experience learning how to forgive, let go, even feel sorry for some of the people that have hurt me big time. Not a piece a cake to do or even go that deep. We don't have to. This life has no rules. Live and die. OR... make it wide. Let all this stuff teach you a better version of YOU! Maybe not try to do it all when you are smack thick in fog. But just becoming more aware. That is the secret. Learning who YOU are. Waking up.

Anger might serve to teach you how to stand up for yourself. So I don't discount it as a wasted emotion. I am once again, just saying it can also be really poisonous. This book is about lifting fog that limits our lives.

Please, if you read this and find that your anger comes up frequently, pay attention. If you want to blame, or you harbor grudges, or you yell to feel better, you are bringing damage to another. They do not deserve it. They might be doing the best they can in that moment to deal with you and your off-brain. There is a chapter ahead on the Toxic life. It too will shine some light into how and why anger can dominate us. Some important things that we actually can do. Lifting fog is no free lunch. There is work. But it happens on a deep cellular level of growth. Little by little, these shifts add up. Becoming a new life and new person.

I want add, I held our sweet Tinkerbell for a long time and apologized over and over ... and never kicked a cat again.

Consider this, if your anger is like a volcano that erupts and spews out angry lava over someone you love, you might feel better afterward. Kinda like waiting and avoiding vomiting and when ya finally get the bug or food out of you, you begin to heal – but, and this is a BIG-ASS BUT... the person that you spewed on, maybe more than once, gets the emotional injury.

The trust level suddenly gets tested and weakened, maybe even begins to imprint that it is their fault or to not trust because of you. I can say from sharing that brief little tidbit about my past, that violence and screaming can stick with you for years. Dare I say, 20-some years? That man will never know what damage happened. Because he was the volcano. A loved-one is not a counselor that is being paid to release emotions at. They are – the loved-one.

This slices both ways. I have heard caregivers yelling at the injured and disabled. I heard it at the TBI conference. I could not believe it. It was when they were out of ear-shot of others, yelling in the hallway "You stupid asshole! Wow!

I know it is really difficult for Dementia partners. Not understanding what is happening to their spouse. Often, by the time the symptoms are a reality, the spouse is exhausted already and may look back and remember how angry they were. The sad part is then of course, remorse and regrets might be the next torture for that spouse or child. Especially if they go to a nursing home and/or die.

If anything I say here - can plant one seed of thought about this fog of anger, then I will be glad I shared.

I am not trying to sound Pollyanna perfect. I am so far from it that I have avoided getting close to many people because I did not want to have them see or feel my foggy pain. Or risk one of my scrambled emotions landing on someone I care about. I preferred the lone wolf approach as a recluse, best I could, until I could heal and resurface. That can have some dangers too.

Each thing I am trying to remember to share in this book delights me in a weird way. Especially putting such a whopper together, and little things like finding a tiny scrap of paper in my brain bonk book that says: Milk in coffee Pot. Anger. Over-flowed the tub. Confrontation. Depression. Whatever I have tried to take note of over these years, seems to be appearing when I need them the most.

While writing this portion of the book, I remembered Christmas 2017, where my dad still was driving locally and took my mom to my brother's for dinner, just 5 acres away. Something happened that is an example of anger and a brain not working correctly anymore.

I was typing along, when the phone rang. It was my brother. It was dark outside. He proceeded to tell me that mom and dad made it over to their house. They all started eating, and things were going fine, but when a wound-up little great-grandson got near Grampa and started back-talking, it didn't go well. Of course excited for a party and gift opening coming next wound-up is pretty normal. But his wound-up energy began to really irritate my dad. I believe he even tried to punch dad in the stomach trying out his Karate. That was not cool.

In this moment, since I have seen dad come unglued quite a few times, (long before mental injuries) I began to tense up at my brother's call. Dad had announced he could not take it and was going home.

My brother, now concerned for dad, was calling to ask if I could run down and check on him. My first thought? Why me?! Why not you ??? Shit.

Anger. Oh boy. Gee thanks! The explosive potential that could have come out of my dad right then instead, opted to take himself home rather than letting circumstances push him over the edge.

I cannot describe how proud I was of my dad. I immediately jumped in the car and went to check. He had stoked the fire, then put himself to bed. (this still chokes me up.) He was still awake as entered his bedroom repeating many times that it was me. He turned on the light and had a guilty, big-eyed concerned look on his face. Immediately telling me he had to leave so he would not get angry. Now this is a fella that has suddenly had days asking who my mom is. While this book is not about brutal Dementia, it is about FOG. But for any of you reading this, Lord knows, Alzhiemers/Dementia is an unkind, cruel disease.

Though my mom and family were upset at dad's behavior, I really let mom know how amazing this was that he took the higher road, in that state of mind. And that she had better NOT lay a guilt trip on him!

During the window of trying to hold on, remember... that person goes through torture. I hope there is some spiritual big lesson for that soul and/or those caring for them. Because it is brutal. But for my dad to be aware of his anger on the evening of me writing, is pretty cool. He could have blown like a volcano but he didn't.

This experience took me back just a year prior when my folks had to live with me for over a month, when my mom's ulcer blew and dad kept getting torrential nosebleeds. I had my hands full 24/7.

At one point in the hospital those first few days, the gang of family sat in the waiting room. It was stuffed full. Everyone discussing mom's condition, worried. I had to handle it carefully with dad. He and I were home alone in my house. His brain was confused and then would get clear. Now splice this in with my own recovery. Yah. I know! And no sleep.

On the morning I was taking him to the hospital he asked if we were going to lose mom? My heart sank and I hugged him hard and said, "NO DAD! In fact, mom is alive because of you. No one else. YOU! You saved her life. They are helping her get strong so she can come home." He was weepy but got ready to go see his wife.

We got to the hospital and after he got to see mom, I left dad in the waiting room with the family for awhile to go get a little breathing space of my own. I returned and the room was hot, stuffy and full of family. I noticed dad's face getting very worried as he listened to the cross-fire conversations going on. He needed a nap and his oxygen.

I vaguely remember hearing someone say that people die from this condition. Suddenly dad's personality changed. Sitting there in his wheel chair and cowboy hat... he looked around at everyone and he began to tell everyone to shut up. They were not doctors and they were talking way too much. Of course no one meant harm but suddenly dad was being looked at like he was an idiot. Including my brothers telling him to calm down, almost scolding him for getting upset. He was afraid. He needed a hug.

Talk about anger... this time it was ME. Suddenly I felt the anger. Protective anger.   It seemed everyone just had forgotten *dad's* condition and it was his frickin' wife! And for them to wonder why would he act like that. HELLO!

I caught some hell following this for reminding them about dad's mental state. I did not apologize. When one family member told me, "You don't bring a stroke patient to the hospital" I had to say, "IT IS HIS WIFE!" I took my wound-up dad and self to the nearest other waiting room. I had to hold him down as he tried to explain himself. I told him it was okay and he did not do anything wrong. Man I was mad.

It took a long time to calm him down. He laid on the tiny sofa, and closed his eyes. Kept sitting back up, over and over. Finally relaxed a bit.   I stepped away, and looked out the hospital window and tears poured and poured in silence. Of all the people to be handling this part, my brain that hates florescent lights, endless talking, stress, and seeing my dad suffer. What a test, not to crack.

All I could think about was little dad on that couch scared, mom in her room trying to get strong and a room full of people down the hall visiting because of mom's blown ulcer. The same people that did not visit mom and dad.   That was the kicker. Somehow hospital visits bring out this weird mentality of good friend, family member (Samaritan) ... to visit the sick. But where do they go when those people go back home? Poof. Invisible.

Trust me, I will not proclaim I had it together on this day.   I also knew that in a few days, I would be bringing BOTH of them home to my house. Little did I know, I would end up in ER twice in a month, during that window.

Anger can be used for all types of directions.   My

favorite visual of blame, I imagine you have heard this, about the pointing to someone else, to take the attention off of your own doings or guilt. Finding fault. Easy to want to blame another when you are trapped in your injury or pain. When you have all your focus on someone else - you don't have to own your own actions. The pointing of the index finger at someone, leaves three fingers pointing back at yourself. Anger is a wicked poison. Read the label. Use with caution. And if over-dosed on someone you care about, apologize. Be bigger than anger. Or brain injury. Use your heart.

"I love you!" He said, then slammed her head -
then he cried and begged her to forgive.
She tried to walk, he insisted they talk -
This became too much to live.

Anger you bastard, you suck out life -
you dump your lava in blame.
A volcano erupting on innocent hearts -
just to pass on your pain.

So to anger, I say this:
"go back and burn in hell,
I choose to take a higher road -
then you - who scream and yell."
LLL

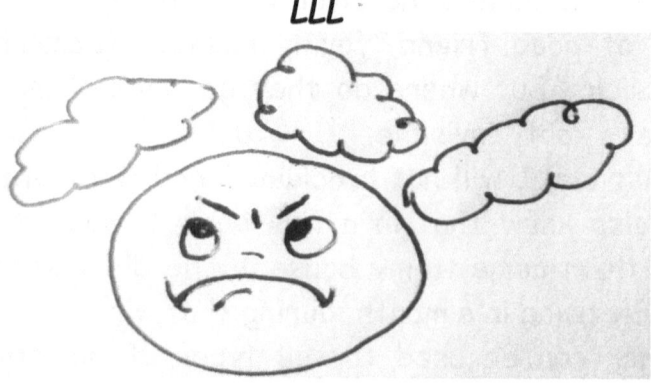

By now, you have to be wondering just how this brain could remember 12-16-20 hits over 10 years. Right? Me too. But as I had mentioned already, there was a first neurologist that I saw, who would not believe I was having seizure episodes, as mentioned, of sudden triple vision and legs would not move, that happened several times a day, lasting almost 6 months. (grrrr yuck grrrr). Very scary.

That doc did however, give me a pearl of advice. I must give credit to Dr. T. here. Otherwise you would not be reading this. She was way above me, and I felt like she thought I was making things up, but, hey, here we are in the NOW. It is all an amazing chain reaction of future GOOD, if we can see our injuries and wounds as opportunity and, HANG IN THERE!

That doc told me to WRITE THINGS DOWN, best I could. Date them. Tell what happened. If it happens again. Tell someone! Reminding you and me... that your brain can swell up to 12 hours after a hit. Now they are finding slow swelling up to 2 weeks, such as mine was after several hits. Oh that pressure. But never enough to drain it, when I was taken to ER. Luckily. It is all so stinkin' scary. I know of two people that died because of this.

Oh my gosh, I know this journey so well. Laying in bed all night after one hit to my forehead, big goose egg, cuddled with my daughter... not wanting to go to sleep because I was afraid she would wake up to a dead mother. Yes. Yuck. Or alone, when my daughter and her daddy went 300 miles south to Oregon to visit grandparents and I had just hit. Hoping this wouldn't be the BIG one, and they would find me face down in a pond or something. Yet, not wanting to burden or scare my elderly parents just down the road. Or complain. Although, I will say, twice, I did contact friends off of Facebook to say, "I hit" just in case. Then, back down the black hole I went.

There is a little bit of both embarrassment and pride that goes with this journey. Through the years, soon as I could lift fog, I would forget the hit, the surgery, the move, the let down of all the record labels, publishing companies - whatever, and try to move on. Try again.

I learned a technique when folk would ask, "How is your head?" "How are you doing?" I would think: "Let's not tell the truth." So I would answer a quick "getting better" and then the technique was, I would ask about YOU! Quick as I could, get the attention off of me. This allowed me to be quiet. It allowed YOU to talk about YOU. You did not know what I was doing. But it just cut me some slack. Made it easier to get through that window.

So for YOU that are reading this, that may remember lengthy visits - I may have used you. LOL! Thank you! I probably remember our talk! Because I tried damn hard to listen, in case I ever saw you again! That is how you live with brain injury and fog. Sometimes in the deep, painful fog, you aren't sure you will wake up.

Another version of the injured brain might be... that the entire world is now only about you. All about your injury. Attending not one, but two of those TBI conferences, (receiving another scholarship in 2016, in which I had a driver) I was amazed how some of us did not want to talk about it, and some, that is ALL they talked about. They could not wait to tell their story. I have had so many hits, I just kinda lumped 'em all together and said "farm accident - not accident(s) if they asked. Some thought I was a caregiver and wondered where my person was! Ha!

As I mentioned, the reason I can share my accidents - is because of that advice from the neurologist. I did not realize I was doing it, but each time I would hit, I "apparently" wrote a little info on a paper and stuffed it in a box or a bag or a pile of papers in my office. It wasn't until my ex husband and I called it quits on the count of pain, while he was moving out, our daughter shared with me, that dad felt maybe mom was losing her mind. Not injured mind, but losing it. While that was killer painful at the time, looking back, I understand.

I have done a whole lotta forgiving for that window of ouch, but that is what actually took me to that Dr. J neurologist. The big brainyologist. To find hope and be told I was NOT nuts. What I found, in getting info ready for him, was my notes. All over the place. That is how I made little stickers on toothpicks and poked 'em in Ms. Thumper, the styrofoam head. All the brief scribbled notes said where I hit, how, the month and year. FYI, much like spell check tryin to add G to my words when I am not looking... should you find things repeated in this book, you will never know if I did this on purpose to make a point, or screwed up. Dang, this is workin' out quite well, me thinks!

As I poked those sticker note dudes in the styrofoam head, I began to cry. What I saw, was like looking at a football player's brain. Or daggum porcupine! All my notes surfaced as if the Universe was helping me. Many notes I had actually written on my computer, trying to describe my condition - over and over. (Boy were those notes hard to read!) Perhaps I was also hoping if something did happen, aneurysm, tumor, something and I died, my notes would be found and people would know I was not making ANY of this up.

Remember, I really wanted you to feel my *brain*. The

random tying together of stuff that to me, has meaning and truth - may not be coming out as you would prefer. Not a perfectly edited book. In perfect order. Too long of chapters for your liking. But how could I? Why would I?

To be authentic in life, you kinda have to stop editing the crap out of your life before you even live it. You have to risk being You. And, even harder, you have to be okay with: *It doesn't matter if you like this writing or me ... at all.* WOW. That one is so hard.

As much as I try to be done with this portion of my life, the only way I can fully heal is to get it out of my head, onto words here, and share. And, if something should happen, that I can no longer write, type or speak - then I will have brought this information, from my perspective, out to the world. And maybe, just maybe, help one person to have hope.

Notes to self:

Dearest Laurie, instead of panic or let fear win:
- This might be school for my soul, take notes
- Be authentic
- Ask to see the truth
- Apologize if I blame another through anger
- Don't worry what others think ... live!
- Forgive where you can.
- Ask to be forgiven.
- Write it down.
- Tell someone if you hit your head.
- It isn't all about you, but don't forget you.
- Don't apologize for your injury or injuries.
- Don't apologize for the life you have lived.
- Relationships are not suppose to be a bill of creating debt, paying payments and interest. Although, some call it karma.
- Try your best to glean something to grow from this condition and experience.

- Let others know that you love em!
- You were given this gift of life, whatcha gonna do with it?
- When you get feeling too sorry for yourself, go help someone else.
- Choose to be as awake to this life as possible. One day that won't be an option. It will be over.
****

Look for the miracles!
If you want a friend, be one.
If you want to know love, then love.
If you want to know forgiveness, then forgive.
If you want truth, speak truth.
If you want trust, then be able to be trusted!

Death will come soon enough, Laurie, so, pick up your bootstraps, and finish this daggum book, without fear, and be open to your next chapter. You might just help another sister or brother in this world and it will be worth all the thumps.

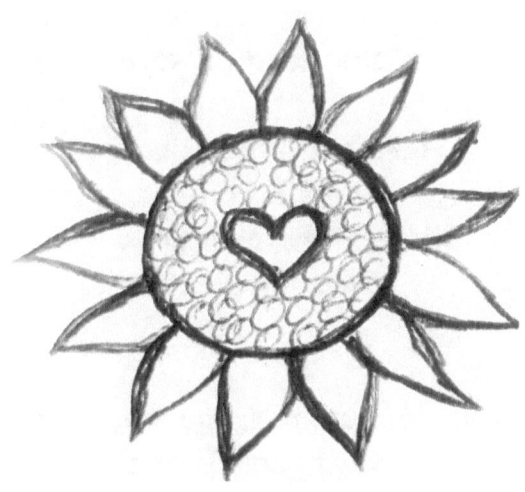

Little head of Styrofoam,
full of toothpicks and many notes.
You represent - a girl alone
Good thing styrofoam floats.

Sayin,' "Go ahead, poke them notes -
Laurie, you are not nuts.
You will use this crazy ride,
to help kick fog in the butt!

For when you thump and thump again -
embarrassed to leave your home,
you see the fog roll out and in -
through the head of styrofoam.

Here's the blessing -
far as I can see
little styrofoam head -
saved my sanity.

You aint nuts girl, you are ... um,
creative! Yah! That's it!
Wink. Wink.

Chapter 11 - Bloomin' Genius

Are some of you reading this and shaking your head at Thumper? Thinking, "I, personally, could/would NEVER hit my head so many times. I am more aware than Laurie that's for sure!" I have to agree with you. You might even say that you would seek medical attention immediately, take the right pill and be on track in no time at all.   YUP YUP YUP, Or - not. Depends on what path of life has brought you to this point in time, reading my book. Maybe it hasn't been hits to the head. Maybe it is early forgetting signs of Dementia, or menopause or gas poisoning, or alcoholism or any brain altering condition.

Maybe you are just curious about brain injury from the inside out, and right this moment have a sharp, quick-witted, speedy texting fingers, and oh-so-smart brain, that has goals and dreams planned. I did.   Suddenly all of those things that we take for granted everyday, like counting by twos, make meals, go to work, drive or unsure where they left their brain - or possibly, maybe dropped into a deep, dark de-pression. Oh boy. This aint the Hallmark channel! Or, maybe it is!

I was a pretty sharp cookie before 2008. Not Einstein, but dag nabbit, common sense was my Webster dictionary of life. Chop wood. Carry water. Or rather, build fence. Write song. Plant farm. Mow lawn. Can vegetables. Pay bills. Drive my folks. Be great mom to daughter. Good wife. Do our taxes. Laugh at funny jokes and movies and recognize myself in the mirror!

While I cannot say I was a know-it-all, jaw-flappin'

talker - I did almost everything myself and common sense and hands-on experience really were my background. I knew somethin'! I still do. It was just that my giddy- up go, done got up and left for awhile, stuck in fog.

Why bother asking for help when you can use a hammer, drill, skill saw, steel fence post pounder, jig saw, plus - balance a check book, make nice meals, grow, harvest and can your produce and talk on a phone. (like everyone else.) HECK YAH! Damn straight. Laurie Lee Lewis, singer-songwriter, farmer, home-school mom. Producer and writer of childrens stories and music videos. Got this. Life is Goooood.

So then, in the simplest act of moving your dining table, and with a rug shampooer - start cleaning the area rug under, bending down to click something into place on the shampooer - standing up full speed to collide with a 40-pound steel hanging lamp. I never did like that damn lamp! Falling back to the ground wondering who just kicked me in the head!

Suddenly in the weeks to follow, I felt dumb as a stump. Like a bad flu had moved in that would not leave. No twinkle in my eyes for several months. Finding myself waking up out on the lawn. Lost. Ah yes. The beginning.

Wow, thinking about this, is hard. Kinda tightens my belly. But, dang it, gonna keep sharing here. That is what I promised God, if God would give me the ability to write forward again on a computer. Most of the time it was jumbled text like this: srue htat ouldw eb so regta. Of course I labored to even type that much not too many years ago. I still often type love, lAurie or aurieL... and have to correct. Funny huh? Not at the time.

I have had to learn so much about this condition. Not dwell, but learn - so that I could disagree when folks would ask, "Why do you keep beating yourself up. What, do you have a death wish, Laurie?" None of it was fun.

I had to recognize that I could not go into loud, chaos

restaurants, or coffee shops with espresso machines, busy loud sports on TV, parties with people yelling loudly cause everyone else is yelling loudly! In fact, I can't wait, even today, to get out of there! But as I have healed I can handle more. Most of the days. Often, I would get the shakes and it exhausted my mind. It also amps up the ringing in my ears.

This is the same brain that when at home, had to forever worry that I had left things on the stove or was over-running the bathtub. And I did. Bloomin' Genius? Huh? "Where de heck is she going with this?" You might ask!

I also can't drink more than maybe a beer and risk that window of "Fog/buzz" that reminds me and feels like what I dealt with for stretches of time - but could not sober up. So you might consider me a very cheap date. Booze Fog. Medicine Fog. Sleep depression Fog. Grief Fog. FOG fog. YUCK!!!!!!

Now, coffee... hmmm, that is a different story. Coffee is my friend. We are pals. It is my one favorite yeehaw in life that does lift some fog when nothing else will. Toss in a smidgin of dark chocolate now and then, this will make a singing farmer smile! To date, in moderation, I feel no need to give up this joy! As long as I include water for hydration too.

There is a lot of talk and positive results about using medical marijuana now for the headaches, anxiety, multi-firing brains... seizures.   To me, that is so cool. I tried it. Didn't help at all. In fact, the fog of a buzz of THC was not cool at all. That stuff wears off when it damn well wants to. You cannot force it. Only tried it once. Yipe, more self-induced brain altering.

The hemp oil for pain, CBC, maybe helped.   Some. The oil itself is proving to be incredible over-all, for health. It is just expensive. But no buzz. No fog.

All this to say, if you are trying to get some brain waves to work, medicating is medicating. It isn't healing. Although, I will say, with Seratonin, being the *happy, positive,* in our brain, that gets severely depleted when we do not sleep or seriously injured or stressed, *some* anti-depressants address that quickly. That is what Melatonin does. Helps people sleep and gives them a lift. So does 5-HTP Triptophan. But really depends on how dark, deep and low you are. You might need something stronger at first.

At least going natural, fish oils, Ginko Biloba, Taurine, Folic Acid, B vitamins, (B-12 in particular), 5-HTP, Ginseng, you are getting a natural source, not something that was tested on a lab rat. It came from the earth. What a concept.

OK this chapter is called Bloomin' Genius because: I have had a few pretty nifty schmifty things happen, while UNDER the influence of self-induced brain altering thumps on hard objects. Whew! Say that really fast!

Now, I realize if you are reading this and are the injured one, you apparently can comprehend what you are reading or listening to. Lucky ducky. I couldn't for several years. I would get so mad at myself. Depending on what area of your brain is injured, will determine the symptoms, quite often. Looking at charts of what area operates our emotions, cognitive and communication skills, balance, etc, it is fascinating. (Oh my gosh, spell check had a hay day with that last sentence!) But, I fixed it, so you think I am a Bloomin' Genius! Baha - Ha!

What isn't always reported with brain injury, at least in my research, is that *genius* that may arrive. Well, at least that NEW spark that wasn't there before.

Some people might say, "he/she is different now." TRUE! We are! And since you cannot fight a brain injury, there is an opportunity for a new level of YOU. If you were in a horrific bicycle, skate board, trampoline, auto, bulls, broncs, quads, ice accident or an athlete of football, hockey, socker, boxer or dirt bike riding and still here, it is worth a woo-hoo-sky! I saw this attending the TBI conferences. I saw the woo-hoo-sky! I saw sorrow, as well. Regret. Struggle. Depression. But so many stories that were shared - all said the same thing: "I see life differently now."

Of course, if we heal, we may forget that wise awakening. It is easy. Kinda like child birth. Some women forget enough to do it all over again. One fella I met could not wait to get back on his skate board, that he had been on with his accident, and to hit the slopes to ski come winter! I remember seeing his wife cringe, but smile.

It is easy after the fog to just jump back in to our old selves. Old patterns. Shoot, I had hit my head many times over the years. Didn't even think about it. Falling off horses. Kitchen cupboards. Tree limbs. Just said ouch and got back to whatever I was doing. But then, came the one that changed everything. The one hit of July 2008 and the many to follow.

Heck, I have a friend who hit her head on the rear view mirror in her car. She might have even considered it a quick bump and thump. However, it changed her for months. It isn't how many times. It seems to have something to do with how it jars the brain. Sends it flying to the other side, floating in that fluid (that protects the brain) and hits your skull from the jarring impact.

Another friend fell, *cracked* his skull, his brain was actually falling out. Horrible. Man, he is a miracle story. There are millions of stories. There are over 1.3 million head injuries reported a year. That's reported. What about all of us that aren't reported?

So how many, if you could ask all those thumpers out there, how many do you suppose would use it as a *wake-up call?* A message to a deeper meaning in life. Perhaps showing that they/we were so busy thinking of the past, the future, goals, survival, relationship drama, anger and so on? Then boom!

When The Fog Lifts, the really thick fog, it is an opportunity to ask WHO AM I NOW?

I have seen very optimistic, religious people that are certain they know the truth about life, purpose, God... who suddenly go very negative. As if God failed them. Read any brain trauma journey, you will probably see a thread that connects us. First, denial. Then blame. Then, burden. Then depression. Then a light. A deeper life. A twinge of fog-lifting. Then more. Inspiration. Gratitude. And then, the **bloomin' genius** arrives. **Purpose awakens**! Well, not all stories. But some!

If we have a clue, suddenly we realize how magnificent we actually are! I don't mean that in any arrogant sense. When our brain starts to heal and we can speak again, walk again, track another again, tie our shoes, it feels like we MUST pay attention. Something BIG is being shown to us. The Bloomin' Genius of appreciating life and opening up to its wonders. Instead of the small, limited, programmed minds that we sometimes become, in our little safety box.

I find it interesting, how stories like a little old grannie or grampa, with Alzheimers, who, perhaps was a devoted Christian, suddenly becomes a swearin' like-a-sailor thief, stealing from the others at the nursing home! Wow! What is that? What does it say about us? Or the meanest S.O.B you'd ever meet - becomes soft and gentle. Are we all wearing *masks of survival*, but don't get to take them off and actually be our true selves in our lifetime?

NOT - that we are swearin' sailors and thieves! Goodness no! I just mean we are being something to fit in. But what is it then, when suddenly the brain injured begins hearing songs, want or can play music, paint, dance, write books, speak in the public, suddenly kinder, more patient, less selfish? Or becomes a humanitarian and sees us all as one big family to protect.

I am not saying we need to bonk our head so we can build a new, better world. I tend to believe the FOG arrives right on our life's journey for a reason. It can mess us up big time. It can win. We can get lost in the fog and never return. But that can happen anyway, even without an injury. Just look at our world of drugs, porn, stealing, murder, hate, diseases, vices of all kinds, medicines, belief systems, politics, money and power.

I want to say something that just filled up my heart, right now. I LOVE YOU. I may not know you or ever meet you, but I love you. I love that you are here. Trying like me, to not just survive. To thrive. To wake up to a deeper meaning of why you are here right NOW. Lifting fog.

I did not have all this information floating between my ears before 2008. Just wax. Shoot, the idea of writing a book about hitting my head, spirituality, growing through injury... ha! Not! In fact, I hoped I would write a book of how daggum successful I became in the music business and how my songs touched the world and helped humanity. Well, I aint dead yet!

For me to take this brain and in time gain big insights, extract HOPE, heal and share this. Zowee! To then sit at a computer, for *forever* and a few days... and do this whole type, edit stuff. A HOLY SHITOLA fit right here! How I set my fingers on the keys and it feels like they start typing faster than my brain is forming the words. It is wild.

That is why I called this Bloomin' Genius! The exciting part for me, in my 50's, I feel like a new life is started. I may be wrong. I might only get til the end of this day. But, at least THIS DAY is cherished!

You know what? YOU are a bloomin' genius! The fact that you are still on the planet. Survived so far. Have an interest in busting through fog to live fully... BRAVO! KUDOS! GIDDY-UP! Shoot, the fact that you are still reading this book. That right there - says everything if you can track my silly, hillbilly writing!

Now, of course to keep it real, if you saw me on a migraine day, where my zippodeedoodah had no zip... and I could barely hold my head up, let alone carry a conversation... I might not be so on fire for the day. But I tell ya, when those skull busting, throbbing, squeezing, nauseating suckas finally leave... PRAISE THE LORD and all that is holy!

A little thump, a tiny bonk
no big deal I say,
heck I do that all the time
I am fine the next day.

But what is this? It is the next day
at least I think it is or was,
just a little thumpy bump
dang my ears have a buzz.

Just a minute, I have the word,
its on the tip of my tongue,
what were we just talking about?
This was easy when I was young.

Are you mad at me today
cuz I canceled again due to pain?
Do you think I make this up?
OH the journey of the injured brain.
LLL

Chapter 12-*ish* –
Foggy Mornings, Clear Skies at Night

Ya like the "ish" on Chapter 12? Somedays are just full-a-ish!

When we aren't sharp, clear thinking or unable to see what might come next - we can consider this foggy. As the day goes by and by night, we might have some clarity. Trusting that each day will bring a little something, encourages us to get up. Try again. Brain injured heads know this one very well. But so does anyone going through ANY trauma.

I am still befuddled as to why we would induce a fog, via drugs and alcohol. Since I have gone through the kind that takes months to lift... it is beyond me. But I guess I did not know that before. We would have less drug users if everyone had a window where they could barely walk, talk, bend. People would appreciate our brains a lot more.

I know quite a few people. All walks of life. Christian, Atheist, Buddhist, Sales Reps., dirt farmers, entertainers, photographers, natural and conventional medical doctors and practitioners, worldly people, life coaches, loggers, mechanics, teachers and the list goes on. I am blessed to call these people friend or family.

Each of us has our own unique perspective of what we are doing here, and why life is. Or maybe never even thought about it, because they are just living, surviving or very into TODAY - aka one day at a time. THE NOW. Which, in reality is what we have.

Starting out with foggy mornings, clear skies at night is about revealing deeper meanings. How our perspective can change from the morning til night... of pert near anything.

Being a songwriter, and watching my writing shift from love songs, country stuff to a more spiritual, uniting healing music, confused a few folks. Wondering what the heck. Who is this new Laurie? If they heard it from someone else, say, Tim McGraw sing: Live like you are dying, or Garth Brooks saying: IF TOMORROW never COMES or Bette Midler: From A Distance etc... that made sense.

I can tell you, going from my, kickin' country to melodic WE ARE ONE, ONE LIGHT, PEACE BEGINS WITH ME, ONE TO ONE enlightened, connected stuff... was NOT an easy birth. Talk about fog. Fog of changing what I was raised on. What I had done for at least 30 years. Furthermore, the obvious part of WILL ANYONE LIKE THIS?

Putting my first CD out called: PEACE BEGINS WITH ME after 911, was a scary process. "Where is the steel guitar and fiddles?" I remember being asked. Risking to grow and change is a real fog buster.

One of the MOST beautiful things that have happened bonking my brain, was slowly, repeat slo-w-ly - not worrying what other people thought. Just record. Just write. And give thanks that I got another song. I can still play instruments and produce music, and so grateful. Gratitude - is a *powerful* fog lifter. It can take foggy mornings into clear skies at night. No matter what. Good ol' Gratitude. Who'da thunk. Sure a lot easier to read it or type it, than live it, right? But it is THE game changer!

Even on an absolutely crappy brain-full-of-pain day, unless I have not slept for 3 days because of a massive pound-er, MOST of the time, I have been able to find something to be grateful for.

Regardless of who we are - where were were born, what

we do, or how we were raised - we all started as gooey little babies. Some of us came out a kickin' and a screamin', some very quiet and looking around, some struggling with a cord around our neck, some came out backward, some were lifted via Cesarian. Some come in drug-filled from drug-using parents. Some are in intensive care. Some are preemies.

How de heck does this have ANYTHING to do with Foggy mornings, clear skies at night?

Well, a baby's vision is not clear when it first comes out. Takes some days to really track where mama is. But instinctively, we have a survival instinct that we must eat, to live. So when milk is provided, while some babies struggle to nurse, most figure it out. Mama or someone is there to feed us and care for us or we would die. We are completely helpless.

When healing from ANY trauma, where fog rolls in, you cannot see clearly, you struggle to take good care of yourself day to day, hourly. Not all of us have someone there to care for us. Depending on the severity of the wounds, we may need help. Be it family, friends or medical - to help us get through a foggy day and maybe, have some clear sky nights telling us: "It will be okay. This too shall pass."

I call this *assurance and a little comfort*. Kinda like my mama would do when I was hurlin' with the flu, in the middle of the night, terrified. She would be calm. She would tell me it would pass. I would get better.

Our society is a little clumsy and maybe even lazy when it comes to comforting another. We don't always know how. So, often times, we avoid them! Except when they are in your home. Sometimes, even then.

I had to heal through injuries that have taken place over the past few years, primarily alone. My daughter was here most of the time, but was busy with high school, her own dramas, and every other weekend with her dad. And as her mama, I did my darnedest not to drag her through my stuff. Trying to show her the optimistic side of injury. But there were times I would crash. Tired of convincing myself that everything would be okay.

When you endure 4 MRIs, doc looking for bleeding or tumors, it gets a little depressing and scary. Even for us optimistic ones.   Or with MRIs, where you wait for the following days for results. Wondering in your fog if this will be the test that changes the course of your life. Or the trip to ER for a CT and they ask if you have eaten in case they have to get you to surgery to put tubes in to drain the fluid.

My daughter and her dad went through so much in the front end of the first couple hits. The crawling on the floor when I would lose my balance. The making dinner and half way through the meal would have to leave the table to go lay on the couch.   The weeping of a lost soul, trapped in my body. Unable to lift the fog. The starring to outer space.   The loss of humor. The frustration of not being able to pay bills, so I taught our daughter how to write checks. It ended up as part of our homeschooling.

The nausea of trying to right in cursive, I would start to shake, unable to connect words. That was horrible.   The inability to count. (which really was hard, because I was very good at basic math.)   The anger of the constant loud ringing in my ears and trying to talk on the phone, to the point of throwing it - as it screwed with my brain. To anxiety of tracking conversations. To sorrow of homeschooling and unable to do a good job, like other mamas were doing. To the eventual divorce. Dealing with my folks dramas and needs. Family misunderstanding me. And so on.

Yet, I can say, many mornings that started with fog in the morning, had clearer skies by night- and this gave me HOPE.   I should include here, that the longer I was upright with spinal fluid, moving, rather than laying my head down and swelling up my eyes, causing all the pressure, generally helped. And, I can count again! Time and gratitude! Yeehaw!

Now - communicating first thing in the morning - well that was another story! Sometimes I would hear my daughter in the morning when she started high school, getting ready for school at 6:30. Being as quiet as possible.

I would drag myself out, bounce off the walls and cupboards but determined to tell her to have a good day. And, that I LOVED HER. Never knowing. Repeat: *Never* knowing. She would sweetly return the love and say, "Now go back to bed mama, you probably only slept a couple hours." Oooh that puts a lump in my throat remembering this. I LOVE YOU CALLIE, (my daughtie!)

Perhaps, that was the best part of when she moved out to spread her wings. She did not have to worry about me. That alone, ironically, helped me. I never wanted anyone else to suffer because of my condition.

When each of us goes through these foggy things, it really is hard to cling to the positive. Especially if you fight it. In which, I did. I fought hard to heal fast as possible or not even healed, get back to what I wanted to do. Or, alone, HAD to do.

Living on a farm, you don't get a lot of breaks to sit and twiddle your thumbs, watching TV and eating chips. Rats and mice find your house. Opossum and raccoon find your chicken pen. High winds, ice, rain, snow comes along and flips or crushes stuff. Trees fall. Firewood needs to be brought in daily through fall, winter and spring. Oh my.

Animals don't give a damn if you have ailments. They expect their hay in the cold, frozen-water winter mornings, stalls cleaned, horse's hooves trimmed. Chickens depend on you. Death happens. Heaven knows I know about this one. Besides 10 years of head bonks, we have buried horses, goat, cats, gerbils, ducks, chickens and loyal dogs. Winter does not wait for you to heal either. Death does not ask your permission if this is a good time for a raccoon to get in and murder chickens or ducks. It happens. And you have to deal with it. And when you live alone and there are bumps in the night, weee!

I say this stuff, not to gross you out, but reality.

FOG happens in FOG!

In some of those moments, man, I admit, tears poured, I felt sorry for myself. I hated putting down my mare, Ester. I cried buckets when our little border collie, Babe got kicked in the head by a miniature horse (we think) and took 3 days to die. That happened the same day as a big event at my farm, for an annual fall food drive. It was nuts! So emotional. Fighting back sad tears and thanking folks for donating food the same day! Sheesh. They probably thought: "Boy she sure is grateful for this donation to feed the hungry!"

I will leave this chapter with this:

Foggy mornings, clear skies at night - this might not be the same day. This expression might mean a week. A month. A year. Several years. Who can barely remember what they had for dinner last night? Right? So, my message here is if you are really trapped in the fog right now, try to breathe in some grace that says: you will have clear skies at night - again.

Believing that something good is coming from your FOG and having gratitude, makes all the difference.

Ooey gooey, so cute and pooey
as lil' babes we arrive from birth -
We learn, we grow, we teach, we sow
And hopefully leave something on earth...

When we exit this journey called life
that stretches our souls to the max -
so that we - can evolve ourselves
to leave in peace, not look back.

The foggy mornings, clear skies at night
with twinkling wisdom stars -
prove that FOG is just more school
as we marvel how we got this far!

Embrace each day as best you can
for life gets shorter with time -
we're here right now – breathe it in
find your balance and rhyme.

LLL

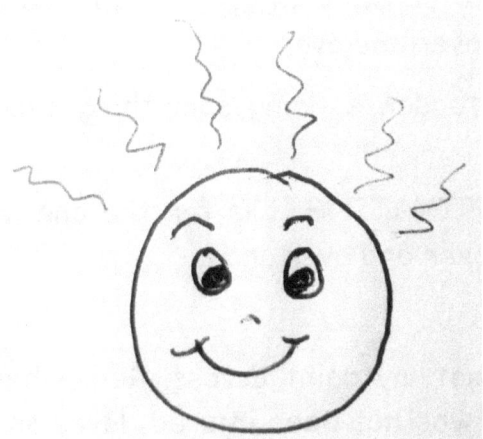

Chapter 13- Pete and Repeat

Pete and Repeat were in a boat. Pete fell out, who was left?

Pete and Repeat were in a boat. Pete fell out, who was left?

"Ya hit yer head again", Laurie?   "How do you do that?" "You should wear a helmet!"

If you feel like you have already read this part in my book, you are right. You did. If you feel like I am repeating myself, correcto mundo!   I am. But for a reason.   A three- part reason:

1. For you to sense what it feels like to hear something over and over and over

2. For you to sense doing something over and over and over

3. How AGGRIVATING it is for the one who has done or heard it over and over and..

OKAY think I got my point across. Remember I am sharing this for anyone who has been injured, loves and/or caregivers for the injured brain and for Dementia, as well.

Not trying to be naughty, smarty pants here. If you are the injured you get this. Another OVER and OVER pattern is the embarrassment of having to ask someone to repeat something because you forgot. Makes you feel pretty dumb. But we are not dumb. We are injured, and on the road to healing. We might even see in between the cracks of life, that others cannot see.

I mentioned before that I would hear my mom so upset at my dad and his post-stroke then Dementia brain, because she had to repeat so many times. Part he could not hear well, part he blocked her voice and part his brain was not running as fast as hers and could not track or retain.

Pick anyone of those and it can really be crappy for the injured.   It is crappy for the one around the injured. Exhausting. I understood my dad's brain and it was exhausting for me! But maybe it teaches a person to slow down their speech. Speak clearly. Make eye contact. Keep sentences brief.

Don't get pissed off if the person doesn't catch up and then, find yourself throwing sarcasm at them like they are dumb. Practice every morsel of patience you have.   IF you don't - you are both going to have a miserable time together! Why would you want to ad salt to their wound?

Over and over.... like Pete and Repeat, only it would go like this: Laurie and Repeat were on her farm just trying to get through another day keeping up with motherhood, farming, bills, groceries, elderly parents, making money, burying animals, writing songs, making CDs, ... Laurie bonked her head again and thick fog moved in. Laurie had to start all over. Who was left? I hope someday that Repeat will move out, and NEVER comes back! Damn free-loader, didn't even pay rent!

The kicker here is, if you are having trouble with retaining information, then if I repeat myself, well heck, it will be all fresh and new to YOU.   So there ya go.

Chapter 14 – Being Kind verses Being Intelligent

In the movie HARVEY, Jimmy Stewart's character sees a 6' 3" tall, white Rabbit named Harvey. A Pooka. Known as a benign but mischievous creature from Celtic mythology who is especially fond of social outcasts. (That part was taken from the movie.) You aren't sure throughout the movie if Jimmy's character is nuts or Harvey is real. At some point he is talking to an employee at an insane asylum, where the family is going to admit him. He begins to share regarding *intelligence*.

In his awesome voice and tone, as only Jimmy Stewart could do, he says; "Years ago my mother used to say to me, she'd say,(licking his lips) "In this world, Elwood, you must be oh so smart or oh so pleasant. Well, for years I was smart. I recommend pleasant. You may quote me."

What I dearly love about that movie, besides the phenomenal acting, is the subtle messages of life, how we are cartoon characters owned by fear, guilt, habit, and programming. Elwood, saw beauty. Gave compliments. Saw the "in between" the cracks of the chaos. Not flustered. Like he Valiumed-out, snorted something, drank or smoked something. Ha, or, maybe ... he hit is his head!

Ellwood opted out of buying into the drama. His big white Pooca friend, Harvey, was like Pinnocio's Jiminy Cricket. A higher self that said, "HEY, enjoy the ride. Be kind. Seek the higher, meaningful road." Good stuff. Good job, Hollywood. Wish we could see more of that, instead of how many ways to kill people, slip sex into family films showing as much as possible without having to change the rating.

Don't ya think it is a pretty good sign when we humans are so eager to absorb our mind in stories of fantasy, zombies, vampires, sci-fi, criminal, romance, violence, porn, whatever – because our own lives are not enough? We want to GO somewhere for awhile. Reality isn't enough. We need to escape and maybe depending on the hunger deep inside, or anger, or wounds, many gravitate to those areas. I admit, I love being taken somewhere in a well-made, inspiring movie.

I have a friend who said he loves dark, painful songs. Especially angry songs. I find this interesting. To me, it seems he hasn't been able to deal with his own anger somehow, so the song let's him feel that pain. My analytical two-bits, there! Subject to be wrong, by the singing farmer!

Publishers and Movie makers are so happy that we will accept their creations of entertainment. Holding us spell-bound to create our reality, for a little while.

Brain-injured heads can easily go there because some brains can't deal with reality. Life makes no sense. Or life is too stressful. But, when the fog lifts, there are some brains, that get a wake-up call and go the other direction. Some brains suddenly want to sniff, taste, smell, see, hear and feel REAL LIFE - not altered reality, as they have been trapped in – in the fog. CLARITY. REAL. ALIVE. PRESENT. BLESSED. Living, laughing, loving. All new, arriving as the fog lifts.

I saw this, in a documentary film by Tom Shadyac, post-concussion, he created a documentary film called: I AM®. All about the above and connectedness. It actually gave me great hope and new inspiration, while in my own fog.

We are in such a liberated time of freedom of expression. Everywhere we turn we are either told we are getting old, so we must spend lots of money on our looks to be accepted, or we are force-fed our political views and if we disagree - we are slime balls.

If we don't attend a particular church with their

particular belief, some pray for us, or invite us for coffee hoping they can convert us - or, if we aren't all eating the same things or aren't the same size or or or...   For being a world that has tried to get away from segregation - if you have had a wake-up call, to a connected humanity as one family... oh boy!

Change may show up, if you or your loved one has had the FOG brain injury, and the fog lifts. You or they may appear to be different people.   Maybe not interested in politics. TV. Or watching movies or news with bashing and violence. Maybe some may be called to help rebuild Mother Earth. Stop wars. Clean up the air. Eat healthy foods and stop being a toxic waste dump site for chemical pharmaceuticals or consuming foods created to grow - no matter how much weed killer has been sprayed on them or the soil.

Uh oh. What if your family is a strong, judgmental, hard right or maybe left *winger*, Or Prozac, Lipitor, Southern Comfort tribe?   And you, or a loved one, suddenly see blessings and pretty auras around flowers! Sees rays of light around trees and people. Sees through the drama. The judgment.   OH NO! AKA: A Wackadoodle - to some! Maybe that person walks out of death and dark slaughtering movies. Passes up the bar to go to a park or walk by the river. Or instead of *prays for another*, they *praise* another, or *both*.

What if you are suddenly very interested in life's journey?   What if you suddenly start writing. Or learn an instrument? Or start painting? Or reveal your true sex preference? Or change your name. Or take chances in life because you realize LIFE IS A GIFT and FEAR AINT GONNA WIN NO MORE. Maybe, just maybe, even make eye contact with each other. More I LOVE YOUs. Live like you are dying. All about: quality. Not quantity.

Brain injury or any life trauma can change the direction of your life. Maybe, if you did sign up on the other side... in spirit form, you made an agreement that said something like: "Hey, God, as human, if I forget completely, and my ego takes over and rules me, could ya send me some reminders? No, really God, I can handle it. I really want a human shot. Looks so fun. Exciting, and I promise - if you send me an experience to shake me off of my path - if it is anything unloving, selfish, mean, whatever... I'll get it. Let's do this.

P.S. You know, God, thinking about this in my little spirit self... if you wake me up from some big experiences... can you then please show me how to use this in the rest of my life? For the highest good? That would be great! But, God, I might need to play a little first. Especially if past-lives is true and I have recycled a few thousand times. Might need a lil time off for good behavior? Just sayin', or rather... askin', and then, if I ever think I am getting too intelligent, arrogant or high-and-mighty, as much as I hate to ask this part - God, can you please send a messenger to me - to humble me back to you?"

Mother Teresa was pretty clear on that in her famous words she left behind:
Three things in human life that are important:
1. The first: be kind.
2. The second: be kind.
3. The third: be kind."

Thanks for her example of a dedicated life work, God. And all the other amazing messengers! You do great work! All we need to do is pay attention to their messages and spread em through our actions. Right? I will leave you the reader with this question? On the scale of 1 – 10, how would you rate your **kindness** these days?

Not bad advice from a tiny lil gal who served "The poorest of poor! I wouldn't have taken that job in Ol' Calcutta. Oy, yoy!

Oh, this chapter gives me the creepolas!. LOL!

Okay... some of you reading this have the amazing ability to know where everything is. Much like the Chapter 10, Notes to self, our brain or literally LIFE NOTES - is where stuff piles up. It can be overwhelming! Yet on the flip, some of you are very organized. While visiting your home or space, you might not actually have the PILE room. You might be clear. Filed. Labeled. Well, here in Laurie-ville, um, NOT.

The very fact, that you are reading an assembled collection of my thoughts, that hopefully makes some sense, well, that is down right amazing to me. Because, organizing anything, when you have had a brain injury or any trauma, or caregiver burn-out - is a struggle! By the way, on care-giver burnout, recently a nurse told me, who works with Dementia/Alzheimers patients, that quite often, the bed next door IS the caregiver! Just thought I would poke that little FYI in here. Just in case, that is YOU!

Back to organizing. Some folk have a meticulously organized house. Business. PERFECTION AURA all around it them. But just about anyone that has gone through fog, somewhere lurking, is a pile. Something you will not address.

I knew that I was at least trying, when I looked at my book shelf one day. The fog had lifted one day giving me some gusto to try to organize, starting with books. I looked at my bookshelf and chuckled. I realized I had 5 *books* on *organizing and simplifying!* HA! Now, ask me if I read one of them? Ah, nope! I chuckled and sighed at the same time. How would I ever push through and clear clutter? Or file and toss. Especially papers! That one is a real stinker. Cuz for me, a writer, there might just be in that heap, one little note, or one spark of inspiration that could become a children's book. A screenplay. A dream I had. A memory for THIS BOOK. A daunting task in my brain. But then, so was making it down to the horse barn to feed, many times!

I am still a pile-r-up-r-r. My barn/workshop will stay organized for 2 weeks till I build an arbor or trellis creation and then the shop seems to explode! Dang rats. Must be them. The horse barn never seems to be clean. Chicken barn, pee yew, but they don't seem to mind. I try to keep up. Someday, this may not be my life. Farming. Critters. But, I realize it is what I have chosen and honestly, simplifying is too complicated, right now.

The house ... well, I have two sets of eyes. One that cannot see if I left a trail of clothes to my bed or from the doorway, the other set will suddenly see it all and nearly have a seizure of confusion and disgust. So then, the two sets, have to have a lil' talk about sanity and say, "You silly goof, just bend over and pick things up and put em where they go! One thangy at a time! Come on Laurie." Do you do this too?

But as life has often done, I will start, then I will check my email, or load my wood box. Answer the phone. Remember I did not pay a bill. And there I go. Distracted.

So, you are probably visualizing a pig-stye messy house. If you stopped by unannounced, you might see a wee bit of this. Things on my table, socks and Buster dawg's fur on the floor, and books scattered around. I do get it all clean and tidy much of the time, so it is probably my imagination, but I have had windows of big mess. I understand it. So if you happen to be on that page, right now... I get it.   Just lock your door or tell drop-in visitors that you are busy so they don't stay and look around, OR ... fake that you are gone. Bahahaha! Or... teach em that mess is okay too! Why not!

I have concluded, since I tend to do many things half-done, that *imperfect perfection* is about being alive, grateful to get another day, and, has to be more important than a dag gum clean house? Right? Right! Besides, when the fog lifts, it is gonna suck up the mess with it, like an inhaling tornado! My house will sparkle and be so organized. No, really!

If it is necessary, business, taxes, bills stuff, that are going to effect you big time, done incorrectly, than, you might need help! Try to find someone to help. That panic of not being able to find something - is a well-ingrained memory for me. Most of the time though, if I remember to take a deep breath, and stay calm, I know it is there and I usually find papers. Usually.

Since I did not read those lovely books on organizing, sitting on my shelf - (partially cuz I do not track reading very long) I have had to find my own way.   Finishing a book or even an article is nearly impossible for me.   Even my favorite subjects of health, farming, spirituality, I just open and take bite sizes to ponder. So it still baffles me that I am writing THIS dude. Considering how many times I have had to read what I wrote - to see if it made any sense at all! Hmm, say now, that sounds a little fog lifting!

I will say, when I have gone to someone's home to stay and it was so tidy, I found myself going home and trying to be a bit more like that.   It felt nice and spacious to see organization.   So, I have tried to copy cat. Pretend I was them for a cleaning spree. Or ask, "How would so and so do this?" Of course the best one that gets me going, which is silly, but hey, cleaner is cleaner, I'll take it: THE COMPANY COMING game.   Power on. Clean. Or toss in a closet. Do you have one of those closets? Or rooms? Shhh, you can tell me, whisper it to me, I won't tell anybody!

You know, admitting this here in print, is REALLY crossing the line. Not only have I told you I have walluped my head over and over, and that I farm, write and record music, and stories, etc... but, that I am also stinkin' messy! OH NO. Am I going to MESSY HELL now? Ah well, I am cold a lot anyway. So fiery pits of warmth would feel nice.

The irony here is with this self-induced pressure of organizing to make life have more elbow room, some resemblance of order – well, if any of you own cats, they will show you something hilarious! If there is a pile PPP-PERFECT! MUST SLEEP ON PILE. YAY! Good job! Don't move pile! I just got on it! Dang! Purrr purrr!

When it was not just me, my daughter and before that, her dad, the 3 of us - that was more piles. More stuff. And I admit, at times of post-concussion, that clutter, mess, dishes, piles... was pure anxiety and I would get very upset at them for not doing their part to clean. Of course they did not understand this need.

My ex-husband was tidy in his own personal space. And his shop. And worked full time. I understood I was at home and it was my job to keep a clean house. But my brain was altered. To just get up and make it to the kitchen, some days was monumental. To try to make coffee and since I love milk in my coffee - suddenly waking up from the fog to see I was actually pouring milk in the coffee pot - where the water goes. Or leaving all the cupboard doors open, perfect to hit my head again. Or bathtub running, or fridge door open, or burning a chicken in the soup pot and filling the whole house with black smoke – or, or, or...

I hated it. Then to struggle to make a meal, and maybe watch a movie while eating and if the two of them did not help clean up, I was livid. (Yah, I hadn't read my own chapter on anger yet, cuz it hadn't been written!) I was wasted. And honestly was mad that they did not try harder to help me. Why should I have to ask? Couldn't they see my scrambled-egg brain struggling? The mess? Well, sure they could. Sure they helped. But, we have to remember, this was not one hit. It was BIG ones. Little Ones. All effecting my being alive.

I would get pissed at my then, husband (always hard to say ex when you are still friends and respect each other.) If we were attempting to have company while I was still in the fog, and suddenly the one who would sit and read magazines on weekends, would suddenly be barking orders out to CLEAN the house, "COMPANY is coming!" While it worked, I did not like that man in that moment. I felt like it should have been happening all along!

After the divorce, it was my daughter and I here for 3 years. She will admit, she had: lazy-ass teen syndrome. Because of the divorce and probably a load of guilt that parents do, (especially my brain) - always wondering if my injuries was the real cause of divorce. I'm sure I coddled and over-compensated as a mom. At least I think. If she was gone, I'd fly around to clean the house best I could, make a meal, spend good time with her. But she knew it.

She realizes it now and how much work it is to keep up a home! She took advantage of it. Fesses up to it now. Good girl, Callie! Probably still can't quite grasp all that mama did, even under the influence of brain-injury. That was her mom. Git'r done. Still is.

I remodeled the house, built stalls in the barn, rearranged the farm. Kept going. Cuz if I sat down too long, the blues might grab me. When I would ask for her help on the farm or house, I would get the grumble. The face. The "poor me daughter" energy. I really dis-liked both that part and having to feel like the bad guy sayin' MOVE YOUR BLOOMIN' ASS DOVER! (I love that line of Audrey

Hepburn's from: My Fair Lady. Sorry. But, its true! No free lunch on a farm, dang it.

Shoot, even as I have been finding windows of time to write this, as most writers will tell you, it isn't sit down for days, sippin' coffee with a bird on the window sill and starrin' at the screen. Oh wait, there is a bird out there actually! Country farm life - is busy. Oh well, keeps my spinal fluids a movin'!

So back to some really cool and groovy ideas, techniques, discoveries that I have found, about this whole organizing issue, challenge, and maybe even a reflection of my life. Messy house. Messy life? Messy mind? Oh gosh. Hmmm. I wonder. Try telling that to Einstein way back when. Or a great painter or sculpture, that created what we regard as brilliant. Their brain could not give a damn if you approved of their house-keeping abilities, they weren't here to IMPRESS us that way. They were here to EXPRESS. Wow. I like that. Think I will reread it myself!

Kinda like these words that I am writing to you right now. I have never thought of this paragraph. I am just touching the keys, with a seed of thought, regarding organizing and the pressures of that. This is what is being written. My dishes aren't done yet. But you are getting to read *this*, cuz I left the pile to write *this*. See? Win/win.

Hey, you 'spose by me just writing this chapter, I will have to go pick up my socks and do the dishes? Maybe, maybe not. Maybe I will go play a song on the piano. So much more FUN! Or take a walk on the farm with my silly border collie, Buster, who makes me laugh. Now Buster dawg.. he knows how to play! Pure bliss and joy!

I want to leave the idea of *imperfect perfection* with you. Cut yourself some slack if you are on the page of piles and mess. If you can trust someone to help you organize schmorganize, perhaps go that route. Take a deep breath and see it clean, visualize that this day will come. But today, if the fog is thick, this too shall pass. Be okay with today.

If you do find you can stay on task, some simple help ideas can be starting with one room. Getting a bag or box for donation and a garbage bag. Hopefully more goes to donation. Or garage sale IF ... it too, does not become THE PILE ROOM. Personal experience with that one!

* Bathroom, organize and toss.
* Linen closet, refold and donate. Bedding, make up ready sets, donate old ones, fold up blankets.
* Dressers, take everything out. Discard ripped and crappy. (Or, keep em and donate the good stuff. Its your life!) Donate if you have too many.

* Closets, it's hard, but removing everything, sorting to bags, placing odds n ends in boxes, write on the edge with a sharpie.
 * Kitchen: one drawer, cupboard at a time. Room to room is a good way. And pacing yourself.   Kitchens are intense because of cupboards, drawers, fridge/freezer, stove, microwave etc.
* Office: another overwhelming space, one file pile at a time! Labels. Toss old papers. File cabinet or box.

ALL of this can cause anxiety and exhaustion but if you can align your brain with: this is part of my medicine and healing, and I can do a little at a time – it is possible to get motivated to organize and simplify.

I write this with all my jokes and piles, but I do say I have made stride. Not there yet.   And really, where is THERE when you get there? Honestly, it might take a complete move before I will really part with some stuff. Easy to just move it to another room. It all takes time. Something I don't have much of these days.

Heck, want to hear something pathetic? That pile room that I mentioned for garage sales, ha, I found myself going through the pile of stuff, and sayin', "Well, hey, I'll be doggone ... lookie there, always wanted that thangy!" Pfft! Yah right!

Well, with a healing brain, we have to cut ourselves a wee bit of slack and laugh! I laugh at my sillies quite a bit. Have cried plenty too.

Just try not to bad mouth YOURSELF. Cutting yourself down for all the things you have NOT done. It DOES NOT help the healing one bit! Maybe even slows it down!

Now, if you have an OCD busy brain living with you - who cannot stand your piles, well, shoot, ask them to GO FOR IT! But have them label things *really well* and run stuff past you before it goes away! The last thing you want to happen is for someone to actually help and when you did not know it, they dumped or donated something important – and you cannot find it. That can be as bad as the dag gum piles!

Piles and piles,

miles and miles.

When I finally see space

Smiles and smiles.

LLL

Here is a big one. Get ready. When the fog lifts on things we never thought about. This one: driving. I am not filtering through this book and chapters to see if it all fits. I am asking my soul to glean what I have learned in the past 10 years healing, and to share.

This one... oooh doggies... this might make a few butt cheeks pucker with reality. Let's just see!

So how is your driving? If you drive? Or maybe you are the passenger, but help the driver! Would you say, you are safe, responsible, courteous? Or, when you get on the road, immediately - you see: *horrible* drivers! Language comes from your lips that you did not know you had when you see: little blue-haired ladies going 30 in a 50, or an old man forgetting that his blinker is on for 5 miles. Or has one foot on the brake and one on the gas? Or cuts you off? Or turns out in front of you from a side road, slower than a slug!

How about this: traffic is so backed up. You left on time or a little late for an appointment or work, and you get some yo yo in front of you, and suddenly you have a few things to say? Even though they cannot hear you!

How are your butt cheeks? Pucker, pucker? Anything hitting on a button here? Hang in there, I am driving us some place!

What is it, about that pinnacle moment... when one gets their license, puts the key in the ignition, turns on the motor, puts it in gear and heads out? One might say it is the rights of passage to drive responsibly to get from A to B. Others might say it is the license to be ... frankly, an *ass*. Ooops. Did I just type ass? Ah, yes.

Now I know a few of you will squirm at this chapter because you are going to be looking smack in a rear-view mirror. While you might be seeing someone tail-gaiting you, a corner of the mirror is lookin' at a part of your face! Are you deciding to turn the page? Ah, but wait, this is about lifting fog, remember?

I love looking at what a dented brain shows you. One thing for absolute I have noticed as I have gone through the fog, is the mentality of drivers. Or, lack of!

You have your slow poke. The tail gaiter. The passer on a corner where you have to slow down. Or pull off. The traffic merger. The bat-out-of-hell car taking a corner coming toward you ... the cigarette in one hand, pop or cell phone in the other (not sure who is driving) or the one I saw typing on a computer, that was sitting on her passenger seat, swerving all over the road. Almost side-swiped me. Or the one who is pretty sure they can drive drunk or high. Or the one who has his bad-ass bass speakers so dang loud that your coffee shakes in its cup holder... even though apparently they cannot hear the dbs inside. ARRRGH! Lil' Pirate talk there!

Here is what we don't know behind our perception of *the ass*: Maybe someone is heading to the hospital, with terrible news. Maybe someone has a baby in the back seat crying and mama is seriously sleep deprived. Maybe someone is tanked up on cold medicines to get to work to keep a roof over their family's head. Maybe someone just broke up with their love and is furious or devastated. Maybe your car is smoking and you are trying to get off the road! FOG comes in many packages.

So why am I picking on DRIVING? Well because it is

one more mirror to hold up about who we are. Our humanity. About having a little grace for another person. And a reflection about self-absorbed mentality. Some impatient drivers might actually be on their way to church! How about that?!

Now, let's put a brain-injured person in a car. Like me. Fog finally lifted after not driving for almost 4 months and hating that someone had to drive me around. Or maybe it is my now, crossed-over dad. Before severe Dementia, post-stroke, (man of the house) 82 years old, still tryin' to do things to be the man to help his wife and go get "milk for ma" about 6 miles away.

If you are one of the listed drivers above, and you were tested by the Department of Motor Vehicles and they were your passenger, but you did not know they were testing you - What would they see and hear? "You idiot! Get out of the way, old man! You should not be driving" or... (gently) "Come on in or maybe, sorry about that or ... there ya go" Kinda like holding a door open for someone. AKA: MANNERS!

At the end of your drive, your passenger asks you to pull over, reveals they have been testing you and gives you your driving grade, as part of how you treat your fellow person on the road of LIFE! So ... (Jeopardy theme music here) do you get an A+ ... or do you get an A-hole +?!

I tell you this, and write about it, because a few of us are still trying to drive on the road of life. And when we get cut off, tail-gated, swore at, passed and scared, we are still trying.

We don't want to be out there. But there is no one in our life to drive us. We want to get our independence back. We have to try. And we aren't always in the best shape. We may have gone out and it is all we can do to get back home. But you know what? We are probably kinder. More apologetic. Because life goes on. Traffic does not wait for you to get better. Nor do bills. Problems. Garbage day.   Empty fridge. Animals. Family. Holidays. Birthdays. Doctor appointments. MRIs. Pharmacies, Death.

Somehow, we have to keep being brave enough to get strong, build our confidence and drive in life, again.

I told this to a dear friend who moved to Washington from California. I totally get how you have to drive fast and defensively on those freeways in California. Or you will get ran over.   But his comment was how horrible the drivers up in the Northwest are! So slow! Until I described my take on drivers.

My friend is awesome. He likes people   He prides himself on the spiritual work he has been doing for years to learn about himself and others. But not til I brought driving into his consciousness, had he even thought about this as a reflection of another part of himself or us. How we treat others, behind the wheel of a car. He loved it. Thanked me. And when I said, next time you come up on a white, dirty Ford Explorer, that is not driving quite the speed for you, or braking at roads to read the signs, remember, "It might be me!" POW. That was it. Lesson learned. Love & peace, man, love and peace! Grin, wink, grin.

This chapter nearly got deleted. But I feel part of this journey, lifting the fog of who we are in patterns, bad habits, complaining, never enough, never catching up, all the stuff - it is also FOG. WE get programmed or duped into beliefs. It too, owns us. So I think I am meant to write this.

WHEN THE FOG LIFTS... this is about LIFE. Not multiple concussions. This is about lifting us up to respect another person and ourselves. Rather than spending precious life energy as fault-finder, complaining. Now is now. And I think, we can choose to make now pretty good! Whether on the phone, calling about a bill and you reach another country or driving along and someone passes you and nearly causes an accident. A deep breath, a lil' gratitude. A little grace.

Maybe, that zooming car just got a call that their little one is in ER. Or daddy had a stroke, or mama is dying, hurry and get here. WE DON'T KNOW. SO why pretend we can. In other words, if we can stop assuming we know someone else's brain, thoughts, actions and feelings... we will make great stride to improve our world. *That* - can lift FOG! WE are in this together. The moment we put the key in the ignition and enter the road of life.

As I told my ol' dad when he was just a bitchin' away one day sayin, "Man, that Guide Meridian road is so damn busy. Cars everywhere. So crowded. I hate it!" (As my dad could do well!)

I hated to pop his soapbox bubble, but after he was done, I said, "Yup dad, it was a gravel road when you were young. But remember something, YOU are part of the traffic too. The crowded road." He grumbled, paused and then... in his sweet, ol' appreciative cowboy manner, replied, "I 'spose yer right Sis."

So to you reading this, if it made yer butt cheeks squirm a little with guilt, here is my Mother Teresa attempt at profound wisdom: Hey you: "WE... *ARE THE TRAFFIC.*"

How are you driving on the big road of life **?**

Time to exit this chapter. I just saw a coffee drive-thru!

Hurry up, hurry up
get out of my way old man -
Can't you see I'm late for work
or I really need the can.

~

Or: Sorry, you are in my way
but the hospital nurse just called -
said hurry if you want to say goodbye
I don't mean to tailgate at all

~

Or: I apologize for my slow car
this is my first day back on the road -
I am nervous but out of groceries
Maybe injured, maybe old.

~

Or: There is a fog that holds my brain
but life must carry on -
so as you pass like a bat out of hell
this aint the autobahn.

~

In fact you might make me have a wreck
because you just must be ahead -
so you risk - both of us
that's how we end up dead.

Chapter 17 - Burden or Blessing

This chapter is hard to write. I might keep it short because it still hurts and since my other chapters have been pretty long-winded. Heck you may have put this book down and shook your head! Hey at least it isn't War and Peace. Oh wait, it kinda is. Finding peace with the war of healing from brain injury.

So, you can imagine, one accident. One event to heal from and ask your family and friends to try to be patient and understand you, right? For the most part, I have stayed a recluse during my big owees. Divorce, miscarriage, brain bonks - I am not into drama so the less others have known, the better, except for what I choose to share, always tagging it with: LIFE IS A GIFT! I don't take it for granted!

In my perspective, why bring others down? Why not wait til your balance is back, eyes aren't so swollen, that you even scare yourself in the mirror! Your speech is clear, you make sense and your smile is back. Once again, shining your light and trying to inspire others. Who wants to see the ugly? The dazed and lost. The depressed? The near to suicidal. Right? Who wants to hear or read that? Well...

BURDEN OR BLESSING... sometimes in your fog, praise the Lord, there will be someone out there to remind you that you are loved. Valued. Worthy. Not the ones that might think you are being a drama queen, using your injuries as an excuse for attention. YUCK. Thank goodness for those who know your pain. It isn't always that best friend, spouse, child or parent. You would think it would be. For me, maybe I have come through so much, and made things happen even during fog, that those close to me forget. I don't blame them. They have their own stuff. But solo healing, as I have referenced to before, can be dangerous... especially if you fall into the black hole.

Since I am not one who asks for help and hides like a wolf while healing from injury, I don't let very many people in. What I have learned in sharing stuff on Facebook, during the decline of dad, mom's medical emergencies and such, beautiful people responded with supportive words. Some family got pissed. Friends "liked or heart loved" but when it came to actually a hug. A call. A meal. The question "Can I do something for you?" The empty, lonely page appeared.

I am learning that this is my doings. More than anything. As mentioned earlier, in my few visits with others during serious foggy times, I would deliberately ask them questions and let them talk. Cutting me some slack from saying anything about my head. My heart. My sadness. My life. Most people would think I have the "bull by the horns" in life (my dad's expression) because I have a lovely farm. Animals that LOVE their mama. Abilities to build things from branches and twigs... (part of my therapy and single, simple – brain, income) lol!

So if you looked at my Facebook photos you would see this happy, shining woman, beaming from her thousands of sunflowers, dahlias, zinnias, produces, miniature horses, my tractor and laughing with my silly border collie. YUP. That's me. That's part of me. And that has been the side I have chosen to share. Rarely the dark side. Asking for help, is hard. Being a blessing or a burden has been the biggest haunt for me during this multiple-bonk journey. Some folk would use it for attention. To me, it was just the opposite.

So when I say BURDEN or BLESSING... I know I am a blessing to some. My mom. Who had to come live with me after dad died, because of her crippling Osteoarthritis and nearly dying of Sepsis. Mom and dad needed my love and help desperately. They were too proud and never asked for help from family. But the daughter sometimes falls into that place where care-giving has no beginning and no end in site. It has been me basically asking family to consider helping them! Which I have caught hell for. No more detail needed there!

Some folk find me inspiring. I have had people tell me that I have been a blessing to them. Inspired by my music and writings and giving heart. But when your brain is foggy, and healing, and you have no idea, after enduring so many hits of what is coming next - that flickery light can almost go out. That is how I sought out materials and agreed with some of the greatest spiritual speakers and authors. Speaking about not letting fear win. Using your gifts and that NOW is what we have. We might remember the past. We might get the future. But NOW... now is it. Each now. The next NOW. Sounds goofy, I know. But it is true.

To some in quantum theory and scientific studies of time - time is never ending, there is not past or future, but lookin' in the mirror, I am pretty dang sure those wrinkles were not there 20 years ago, so something is happening with time! LOL!

Have you asked yourself if you feel like a BURDEN or BLESSING? Would you comfortably ask another for help? Or do you hate to burden them? Do you feel like you are a blessing when people are around you? Or, what are you doing with your life to bless others? Hard questions.

For me, the biggest burden was with my daughter and her dad. Daily feeling like I was not a good mom or good wife. I was altered. A real drag. That experience weighed heavier than most other big oweees I have endured. It nailed my self-esteem. To this day, I have a twinge from a few times – when the going got so foggy tough. But I am workin' on letting it go!

I know it gave them an opportunity to grow and learn about this condition. For the most part, they get a A+. In fact, when the divorce finally happened, I felt good. I felt like I released my ex-husband from a responsibility. A burden. No longer would he have to deal with my good day/bad day stuff. My daughter continued to live with me. And our lives were better. Just releasing one strong personality from our home, helped. Not easy. He was my rock. He knew all about me. And, my protector. That was much harder to let go of, on the tight rope, that was so shaky, than any money or stability.

Not too many job openings out there for a single mom on small budget with multiple concussion history, frequent headaches and extremely sensitive to our noisy, over-lit world. Again, burden or blessing? My biggest prayer was that I taught them both this little something about life:

Don't get stuck in your head. Try to come from your heart. Because one day, the head might be altered. Not so smart. Not so analytical. Not so philosophical. But the heart, the heart can feel. Endure. Have empathy. Compassion. LOVE. And that, to me, is far more valuable than a smart brain.

All the knowledge in the world is wonderful. But I am here to say, one big thump to that melon on our shoulders - where you cannot track another person's conversation or keep your eyes on a page or write in a straight line, or count by 2's or times... all of that can go away. For a little while, or a long while. But the heart - it can open wider than we ever imagined! There is no limit to how much the heart can love.

As for burden or blessing... When the fog lifts... we all realize we are blessings. Just by being brave enough to share our hearts, even if its about our brain!

I am so sorry what you endure
trying to love me this way -
I feel like a burden with fog so thick
I know it will go away.
And then I promise to make up time
for all we lost in the past -
And be a blessing in your life
good memories to last and last.
LLL

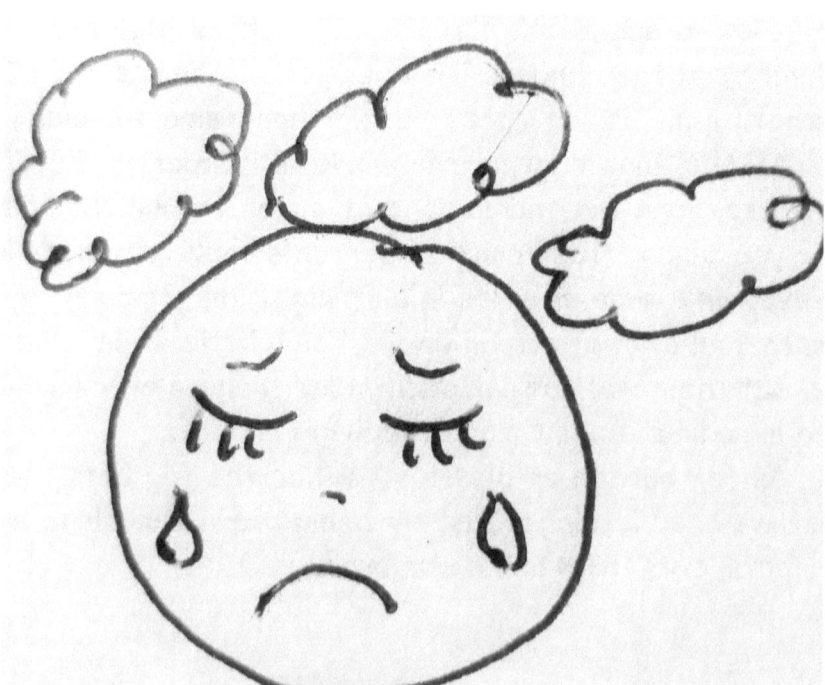

Chapter 18 - Bizarrisms

Because so much of this has been painful for me to go through journal entries, notes on paper, to bring symptoms of head injury to you... I decided just to write out some of the wacky bizarre side effects of some of the few hits. They may not make exact sense to you reading them. They certainly did not while I was living them, and a few, now and then are still here.

This way, I can say I followed through on this part. That's me. Do my best. So I can let it go. Get on with the living, that I need to do, and share, best I can.

Ringing in the ears - constant.

Feel of a hair on eye lids for months

spiders crawling on all over my head

the feeling of hot oil or blood running up and down left side of my face

triple vision episodes where room rocks and legs won't move

brain zaps

eye zaps

eye lids swollen big.

wiggly waves on the sides of my vision like someone is waving their arms.

low ohm train deep vibration in base of skull when I lay down

cat thumps and cotton balls. The ability to hear the most minute sound. Would send an shock wave sensation through my head.

Of course time and memory. Unsure if that was yesterday or still to come.

de`ja`vu – repeating occurrences

the rope pullin' you over and down to the left or right
walk like a duck,
talk like a drunk or stutter
head pounds so hard your head moves on the pillow
songs and movies in my sleep. Cannot shut them off. Complete
movies. Complete songs.
Hiding and recluse behavior
impatient and angry with unkindness and laziness
fingers don't like to do small work.
Such huge effort to do tiny things
seeing 20 projects at once, not doing any. Overwhelmed
crying easily.
Unable to laugh for periods of time. No humor.
Everything funny for periods of time.
Ready to "go home" giving up
going from zero in the AM to 60 in the PM
Not wanting to go to bed and have to start all over again
headaches for weeks, not hours or days...
hating the phone
lost on the farm, finding myself standing in the middle with a
hoe or shovel
attention disorder... start this, end up with that.
Milk in the coffee pot
forgetting to shut off stove, car, bathtub,
burning up pots on the stove
unable to handle panic, fear, causing seizures.
Fearless at times. Climbing high ladders. Crawling under
tractor. ALONE, so alone.
Unable to handle busyness, loud sounds, loud laughter.
Not interested in talking about religion or faith
very interested in talking about both
where did the day go. What day is it. What month?
Paying bills, bouncing checks.
Numb face

Obsessing on a single thought
super sensitive to what others thought?
Didn't give a damn what others thought!
Could not get dirty enough in the garden.
What concussion?
When?
Falling over, bruised all the time.
Spacial awareness gone?
I can. I can't. I will. I won't.
How did I record that?
Did I write that?
Blurt and hug I love you.
Grieving deeply at death of animals
Could see people's pain aura around them
seeing life as a joke
seeing life as a gift
forgetting to eat.
Where did I just go?
Will I remember you tomorrow?
What is your name?
Who is that in the mirror?
Who will love me like this?
Am I crazy?
Be brave or run like hell.
Don't run! You pay the price when you run or pound. Walk away
quickly!
Oh no, here comes the whiner!
Oh no, here comes the long-winded.
Oh no, here comes the teacher. Or corrector.
Oh no... did I make any sense at all?
Is this real?
Is this true?
I can't do this anymore.
I am so grateful to be alive.

Am I crazy?
Dented head.
Am I nuts?
Alive, not dead.

I still see beauty.
I hear the songbird,
But hitting so much
This is absurd.

Really head?
Must you get in the way?
Leaving me bizarrisms
explaining my day.

The fog lifts right?
When it does will I look?
Hell ya man
I'm writing this book!
LLL

Chapter 19 - Nobody LUBBS ME

When my daughter was around 2, with all the drama of *being* 2, she was happy part of the day, then would get tired, grouchy, have a melt down and fall asleep. One particular moment in time, life was just *owee rough, at 2 stuff*, crying, unhappy, she sat up from a big waaah and said, "Nobody *lubbs* me." What could a mama do? The sad little face. Lip out. Big drippy tears from huge, melt-your-heart, round blue eyes. I scooped her up and said, "Mama loves you, SO SO MUCH, so does your Spottie!" Big hugs and kissies followed, and in no time at all, she was passed out on the couch with her stuffed dalmatian puppy dog, Spottie. She survived.

Most of us, at one time or another, have felt that NOBODY LUBBED US. Or we did not know how to ask for a hug. Appearing needy. Or felt very alone.

When the brain isn't working right, it can push buttons that we didn't even know existed. For me, it was hiding. Not answering the phone or the door. Mostly because my eyes were sometimes swelled. My balance was so wacky. During the thick fog, I did not know what day or time it was. I was trapped in an injured brain. And life did not make sense. Not wanting others to see or hear me as I was, while I knew people cared, I just avoided them.

Not long ago, in finally speaking my heart to a long-time friend, I shared that I really needed that friendship when my dad died. She said, "You want to be heard, but not seen,

Laurie." Referring to me posting my journey on Facebook. It wasn't true. I wanted someone who had known me forever to make an effort to tell me they were thinking about me. *Privately.* Not me being the first to reach out and keep a relationship alive. As I tend to do. Instead of "liking" my post on Facebook. While that is a nice way to share things, there is a mental disconnect. People forget that it is just words. It is not physical touch. Real calls. Real connection. Inviting for lunch. Asking if you need anything?

Becoming full time caregiver to my mom, suddenly, both she and I have felt the disconnect. For me, perhaps much more because she is getting my love. My care. But no one helping me. This is a present fog for me. Writing this book has actually been a sanity retainer, during this wacky chapter of life.

We think we are special in someone's life. But then, you might be in the same room and recognize an awkward, weird vibe if you have been posting on social media. Like, "Hey, I already "*liked* you or sent you a *heart* on Facebook, I don't need to come up and actually give you a hug." I am not saying this is standard reaction, just something I have noticed. So instead of heart connection we have social network connection. A piss-poor, watered-down version of good ol' heart to heart love *relationship* - if you ask me. Or, even if ya don't! Hehe!

My foggy windows of pain worked fine while I was married. I had my rock husband and incredible daughter. The first 5 years of the injuries. But when I became single in early 2012, and still not in very good shape, it was the first time I really had to look at brain injury and love. The idea of ever loving someone again was terrifying. Not because I did not think my heart could still love, but never sure what my mind might do. My biggest fear naturally, was that I would begin to care for someone, and either hit again or have some neurological issues return. Or, they would ask too much of me.

At the end of 2012, fall, a high school class mate, was moving from the east side of Washington over to the west, our side. He needed a place to park his 5th wheel and board horses for awhile, as he figured out where he was going to live. While hesitant, I agreed that he could park at my farm.

For 6 months, it was so nice to have him here. Kind, caring and strong! So good to my daughter and I. It was the first idea of maybe being loved again. But intuition entered for me, and while a light romance had barely begun, I asked for us to return back to friends. In which, he has continued to be a very strong rock for me. It was the first good, bad and confusing experience of considering love again. Holding the hand of a good man. Good that it was nice to be appreciated. Bad that if things did not work out, I might hurt someone. Never my intentions. Our dear friend moved off the farm in the spring of 2013. Now happily married.

My daughter saw a Farmer's Only ad on TV and suggested I put my profile up. This really scared me. But it kinda made sense to maybe meet another farmer. So I made a page. I even shared that I had had concussion stuff. Did not say how many. Wanted some chance of an email or two!

To my surprise, apparently from my honest way of writing about my life, I got tons of emails. Overwhelming. I think I lasted a week or two.   During that time, I answered a few emails but mostly deleted them.   One profile stood out. A gentle appearing soul. But it really made no sense to write to him. He was living in Illinois, moving to Alaska. But I liked what he wrote and he had such a gentle smile. I braved up and said hi.   Turned out this man wasn't sure if Alaska was the right place but was ready for a move. We exchanged emails, I baled off of Farmer's Only and we talked about meeting if he was to ever come up through Washington, en-route to Alaska.

As the possibility got closer for him to travel, I chickened out. I had hit my head again and just could not see myself meeting him. I had massive headaches and horrible balance again. Dang fog had moved back in. So, I said no, and suggested pen pal friends.

2013 came and went. Feb. of 2014, my dad had his Stroke, so life changed drastically again. Later that Spring, I braved up again and went on Match.com. Corresponded a bit. Chatted with a man living in Alaska. He was interested in moving to Washington to be closer to his children near Salem, OR. For months we corresponded. Seemed pretty cool. He ended up moving in the fall with hopes that we would be right for each other. As soon as we met, while I really cared for him, I knew we weren't *it*.

In helping move some things I had, that he could use in an apartment he rented, I clobbered my head on a 2 x 6 beam when stepping full speed up into my truck. Boom. It dropped me down to my knees. My intention was to have the truck loaded and surprise him with all the cool stuff. The surprise was on me. HOLY MOLY! I did not fair well from this hit. That experience kinda ended my faith in online dating, as well.

Then fall 2015, feeling stronger, I decided to try Farmer's Only, one more time. Met a lovely man who logged with draft horses. Instant connection. Mostly because of my admiration for what he did. My grandpa was the only man that I knew who had logged with his big Belgians. What felt like instant love, had to find reality. Took a couple months and suddenly I was clear that this was not the right relationship. Again, a beautiful soul. Wonderful heart. Just did not feel right. It also scared me about my future. I certainly had no intentions of hurting men! But I wanted to be loved and love too.

Every now and then, I would get a little hello email, from Illinois. Which always made me smile. He called me the Little Red Washington apple. The man I would never meet. But it felt good to know he was "out there". A gentle soul.

I farmed. Helped my folks. Dad got stronger. My head was healing. Got my daughter through 2016, of graduating high school and the ol' brain seemed to be doing better. I would still get some pretty long migraine windows. 3-4 days. Or balance would go wonky for no reason. But no hits since Nov. 2015! WOWEE! Happy Laurie.

Right about the time my daughter was graduating, I tried one more time on a different dating site. This time, I met someone a far cry from farming. A fantastic comedian. We met and it was so fun to laugh. He said I was as fast as he was with my humor. Even my daughter noticed how fast my brain seemed to be working.

It was lovely. Except, he was not divorced yet. It kept getting delayed.   And he had to travel around the world for work on cruise ships. Those two combined - took a bit for me, but I finally remembered why I wanted to love and be loved. To actually be together!   Farm together. Grow old, if possible, together. So I ended the relationship. Pretty much validating that was it. LOVE and LAURIE was done. It wasn't that NOBODY LUBBED ME. They did! They all did!

It was that I did not trust my head or heart anymore. 4 lovely men. All willing to try to love me. And I ended any future with them. Not just fear. Some deep knowing that we were not the right match. I certainly was not the best brain out there to love. Pushed too hard, too much demanded of me, any signs of possessiveness, jealousy, or the professor correcting – would tighten my brain and heart.   Still, that haunting idea of hurting anyone or my own heart anymore. No. No way.

2016 was winding down on the farm. September was big for me. I had written the song,   WHO WILL FEED THE

HUNGRY, did the food drive and welcoming a calm fall.

Instead, this is when I got a call, the 5 A.M., from my terrified dad about mom's blown ulcer, how he saved her life, and her long road to recovery.

I shared earlier, that following her hospital stay, both my folks then came to stay with me for a month. I gave mom my room. She was so weak that she spent the month on the couch during the day, then barely getting to my bed at night with a walker. Somewhere in there, as I have written in previous pages, my dad had to go to ER via an aid car, for a torrential nosebleed. He had his nose packed with a balloon. Which was horrible! Having to help your post-stroke, terrified daddy, during that ordeal, blood everywhere, I tell ya. Then, mom had to go a few weeks later for vomiting. It was nuts.

Needless to say, for 40 days, I ran. I stressed. I did not eat well. But they were getting stronger. Some family and neighbors helped a little - when they could. Letting me leave for an hour or two. But it all caught up and on the 40th day. I asked my aunt to please take them on an outing. I was desperate. She did. She saw. Soon as they left, I tried to sleep. But could barely breathe. I was taken in the aid car to ER with chest pains. The ER people looked pretty shocked. They had been out 3 times already for mom and dad. Here, they found a wiped out daughter. The doc said, "Honey you have to breathe. You are holding your breath." No kidding! I replied, "It's just easier to breathe out."

I repeated this story about "October" because of LOVE. And, caregiver burn-out.

Is was on one particularly stressful evening, coming from my dad's room, helping him with the recent horrible nose packing that made him moan with pain night after night, and running to keep my mom eating and administering medicines... I got what was suppose to be a joke text from the funny comedian man. I suppose I still held a tiny flicker of hope for us. But this text blew out that spark. He was returning home on a plane, a few bloody Marys later... (sounds like a country song!)

The out-of-the-blue text showed him with a lovely girl joking, "Hey, meet my new best friend from Bellevue!" While any other time this might have been cute, this particular night, in my exhausted and numb brain, post-ER visit, that was all it took to say: "NO MORE." I really felt angry that something like that had to come in, when I needed something loving to tell me things were going to be okay. Not a joke. I think I finally said that I did not get the punchline, this time.

I had gone in my back room and cried. From dumb text, to my dad's condition, to my mom's ulcer and her Osteo pain... I just cried and cried. Maybe 30 minutes later, I heard my phone buzz again and saw a text. I had to clear my focus, to see that it was *not* the comedian. It was Illinois Michael. Saying hello and politely just checking on how I was doing. I was stunned. Of all times!

No intention of responding to Michael with this sudden heavy load of my life, something made me text back, telling him what was happening. Once again, even the remote thought of love, especially long distance, did not spark. But I needed a friend. So, suddenly I had one.

Michael shared that he was very heart-broken when I chickened out of meeting him the two years prior. He truly did not understand to the extent of my brain injury stuff. Mostly because I did not tell all, back then. He shared he had also gone through a rough year. A heart attack. Kinda put us in similar space. This time, I had nothing to lose. He was far away. Most likely would stay far away. But a good friend would be wonderful.

Still in Illinois, Michael was heading to Ukraine for over a month to visit his son through November and part of December. Suddenly, I had this wonderful corresponding

145

going on in Ukraine, with a country boy. It helped the fog.

Something magical unfolded during that month. So much so, we knew we had to meet. Not sure what we would find upon meeting, but I decided to get a ticket and fly to Illinois mid-Dec. For a week. Mom thought I was nuts. Well? Damn close! My folks were back in their home, and the window was right.

You may be asking yourself about now, "Geez, why the heck is Laurie talking about relationships, dating, and so on? Thought this was a brain injury book." YUP and NOPE. It is about the broken part of us trying to fit into life. The world. Real stuff that still comes to us whether we are healed or not. And, how it may not end the way we wanted or hoped for. But we show up and try. Lifting fog. Growing.

The main reason WHEN THE FOG LIFTS is finally making it to book form for you to read, after a 10-year journey, is because of Michael and the promise to my dad, that I would try to talk about this stuff. I knew, the more and more I tried to share with Michael about my journey, the weirder I sounded! Yet, I could not hide my injuries. My past. I wanted to let down my guard to him, to trust. To truly let him see me AS -IS!   So, I said I would write this book, he could read it and if he ever forgot who he was loving, he could read it again!

That was a long way around NOBODY LUBBS me. Turns out, an Illinois country boy moved to my farm and stayed for 18 months. He ended up being the biggest blessing to my folks and me. Primarily to dad. A few blips along the way shifted us back to friendship only. The great blessing was that he was there for dad til his last day. They loved each other very much. Dad died August 3rd 9 A.M. and Michael left for Illinois at 7 P.M. I can't explain that window. Other than blessed and blasted with emotion.

I wasn't sure if it was worth even sharing this part of the story, but I think it is. It is all about love. Amazing love.

That powerful thing that has given this woman the drive, to survive and thrive - through multiple brain injuries! We never know what blessings of love are waiting right there, but we will see them, if we believe and hold faith, that sometimes we can only see ... When The Fog Lifts.

Will I ever LUBB again? Will love enfold me and not ask questions? That would be lovely. Even though, I realize by sharing all of this, it might scare the crap out of some fellas, but it might amaze a few others. WHO KNOWS! We'll see!

If I were a man, would I lubb ME? Would I be enough heart, even if the brain sometimes has glitches? Or even bigger... could I love a man ... that had over a dozen concussions! Dang, I love asking painful questions! Talk about making your OWN butt cheeks pucker with discomfort. This moment, I cannot answer, but completely understand if one said, "No."

To my grown, little daughtie, Callie,
Thank you for lubbing mama through all of this and giving
me your childhood dramatic story, to write that chapter.
I LUBB YOU always and forever, from either side of the
thin veil of life. If something happens to mama, no
worries, you will see me in the butterflies, dirt,
sunflowers and songbirds... and, leprechauns, tryin' to
steal yer gold! Ai!

I AM YOUR MIGRAINE

Your going along fine, having a great day -
when I decide to stop by -
I knock on your brain - send the first pang
hmm, no answer, I'll poke at your eyes.

I start to grow, welcomed, I am not
I force your eyes and you strain -
sounds and light are your enemy now
yes, I - am YOUR migraine.

You try to ignore me, pop some pills fast
and attempt to go on with your day -
no one knows what I am doing to you
as your world goes from color to gray.

Then I hit, full blown at last
to bed you go in consumed pain,
I win again, you poor little thing
yes, I am YOUR migraine.

Oh, you think you are alone -
in this darkness that gets worse with light?
Oh no - my pet, we are many
we can control you - day and night.

Why some brains and not others?
That's a mystery we'll let remain
as for now - I like you best.
Yes, I am YOUR migraine.
LLL

Chapter 20 - Thin Ice

Again, for those of you who are taking the time to read my journey, thus far, I thank you. We are really never alone, but when the injury is between your ears, sitting on your shoulders, it can certainly feel that way.

My fingers seem to want to write about something that pendulums between ego and low self esteem. Calling this chapter Thin ice. Most all of us probably have some memory of where we did too much or said too much. Went over the balance line. At least I assume you have this experience in your bank account of life. If not, holy moly, you and Jesus are amazing.

Thin ice is what we walk on - when we risk. When we kinda, sorta feel confident to try to say or do something. Not completely sure. Ever literally walked on thin ice? I learned something when I was a youngin' about crossing over ponds and frozen water that was questionable. If you softened your step, bent your knees slightly, you could shift the load of weight. Not all coming down hard kerthump in one spot, potentially cracking the ice. Same with slipping. Your center of gravity is different with slightly bent knees. Less likely to fall.

Sadly, I am editing this chapter only weeks after my own neighbor tried to save his old dog, on his big frozen pond. Not only did he fall in, his good friend tried to save him and went down as well. And then, the younger of the two dogs jumped as well. All 3 were drowned when the ice broke.

Shocking to us all.

When fog rolls in, we have to slow down, which is the same as ice. Driving on ice, if you slam on the brakes you go into a spin. You have to learn to turn into the spin. All counter intuitive to what we know. There is a forced slow down or softening. If you grip the steering wheel hard, it is easy to over-steer. Light hands, can often save a wreck! In essence, soften and go-with-the-flow.

Thin ice can be very dangerous. We have to use some common sense and discernment when crossing. Even just a driveway. Sharing this book with you, about my many head injuries is a bit of that ice. Particularly the fact that I am letting you into my world. Setting you up to now judge, believe or not believe me, shake your head at the level of writing, editing or lack of, or bend and soften and realize I am sharing many peoples' stories via my version. That is what connects us.

I am always more impressed with a motivational or spiritual speaker that tells some of the ikkies of his/her life. Their challenges. Their ego. The thin ice they crossed. Their lessons. Not just the professional scholarly book worm - who can tell me what to do, but has never done it themselves.

As I have mentioned, I have mostly lived alone, working my farm, feeding animals, being just a couples seconds from my elderly parents and honestly feeling like I could never catch up. Always more to do. But one of the biggest repeated lessons of all my head injuries was, being in a rush, thinking elsewhere. Not present. Ker-THUMP!

Winter 2017, we got hit early with snow. A bit unusual for Northwest Washington. The snow mostly melted but then temperatures dropped and brought horrible icy roads, driveways and car accidents. I hunkered down and stayed home as long as I could. I learned my brain, and sliding was absolutely horrible. My brain doesn't snap back with balance very well. So a quick slide in my car, starts me shaking. The brain searches and reaches for stability and a constant. For my brain, sliding and messing with it - stunk!

With my driveway completely iced over with a thin layer, I almost found out the hard way when crossing it in the dark to go lock my dear chickens, in their little house. I got about half way across and slipped, nearly doing the splits! Somehow I stayed upright.

I could not stay there frozen in fear all night, so opted to scoot in teeny weeny steps across. I locked up the girls, and repeated going back across. Scarier yet when in the dark. The vision that really shook me up when I finally got back to the house was the reality of living alone. IF I would have fallen and cracked my head on the ice, no one would have ever known. Perhaps 'til the following day or two. I hated this vulnerable feeling. This stuff you have to do, but is high risk. Same with carrying buckets of water down to my horse barn, due to deeply frozen water. They counted on me. Even with a balanced, healthy head, we can fall on thin ice.

From crazy things like this, I have had to learn either you let your critters suffer, ask for help, or do it yourself. This is just one little challenge. On the farm, there are many, any given day. But also an incredible life for a somewhat recluse like me.

Thin ice reminds us much like fog: caution. Wherever your brain is, do your best to get back into NOW. Pay attention. Be mindfully present! I had many trips back and forth out to the barns during winter storms. Knock on wood, I am still upright! Well, not as I type this. I am on my lazy butt, sippin' tea and munchin' a cookie. Woohoo!

Thoughts, words, actions, all can require mindfulness. Otherwise, you might bust through the ice, slip on the ice, land on yer ass and find a whole different level of ouch/injury fog awaiting! Hey that was fun to type!

Now, if you are reading this from sunny, warm Hawaii, you might be chuckling at the whole ice reference. In that case, we might have to talk about banana peelings or falling coconuts!

Dearest ice, your a pain in the ass
I prefer you - inside my glass -
sippin and ginnin and havin fun,
not slippin and swearin - give me the sun.

Winter storms with dangerous ground
its enough each day - just to get around -
add ice to fog of a struggling brain
dangerous ice, you're such a pain!

LLL

Chapter 21 - Saying No. Oh No!

Now for any of you super achievers - who host holidays, entertain friends, coordinate reunions, or committed work - anything that requires YOU to say: "no" ... may feel like you will break. Something terrible will happen if you *don't*: host a birthday, attend a wedding, bring food to a reunion, work over-time, volunteer, attend church, be super soccer mom and so on.

When you are injured, one more thing might be all it takes to put you over the line of anxiety. I know this journey so well, spanning a decade of parties, holidays, commitments to music etc. The calender itself could make my stomach quiver just trying to recognize dates, weeks, months. Committing to something "Out there" with the big WHAT IF, looming. What if headaches come, balance is off, slurred speech, mega fog? What will I do? Bigger the commitment, bigger the stress.

How I have been able to know about my healing progress, was when I would start making plans for "tomorrow and beyond" like singing at a special banquet for Cancer research or buying a plane ticket to travel. HUGE! And while I might have to stew over my schedule more than some, and work backward with time, it is my way to help me be more prepared, so I can relax a bit, and go more with the flow - when I need to.

Traveling can be stressful no matter how you slice it or what you have gone through. I avoided it as much as possible.

Fear had a pretty good hand-hold on my confidence after each hit. Rattled me, then took my sense of reality and altered it. Ddddamn it. So adding things on to it, like events and such, seemed crazy-making to me. However, as much as I tried to avoid putting myself out there, things like humanitarian projects would pop up. And I was able to dive in, from my heart more than my head. And do some amazing things.

Saying no, to a big-eyed daughter wanting to go to a movie or carnival or having to stay home, and send her with her dad or friends instead, was painful. I felt like I was missing out, but knew I would pay a price trying too hard, rather than say no.

I have talked to a lot of people about this subject. Mamas know no boundaries it seems. We are super heroes... expected to do it all. Clean house, good kids, laundry, bills, groceries, meals, yard, parents, decision making, school activities and so on... trying to keep your sanity while your brain is already scrambled... oolala, this can really weigh heavily. Disappointing family and friends. Or so you think.

I cannot say I was a champ here. I said no where I could. I did too much and paid the price. I challenged myself in altered thinking, then regretted committing to stuff. Tie that together with poor sleep, unable to remember what you committed to, I had to deal with a few panic-strickened moments. But, I got through it!

Luckily I would turn to my daughter and her dad during the earlier injuries and give them some of the load. They were, for the most part, very good about this. It makes such a difference when you have someone you can just be okay, or not being okay.

If you are in a place where you are being asked to do things you know are just not possible or cause huge anxiety, that will trickle down into everything else- that's where NO should be used. If you are still healing, try to say no. Try to be okay with putting your needs out there as a priority. Especially when you are just a few days out from injury.

You may commit to something but aren't thinking correctly. I would suggest you even tell the person asking, "I need to get back to you on that." Or tell them about your head injury! Saying no, when you are in the fog, is OKAY! Try... to remember to write things down! I had lists about my lists.

Saying no is hard. I am still working on this. I admire those of you who can. If you are good at this, I need to read YOUR book!

Like... Oh my gosh... did, she, like, say... NO? And, like, oh my gosh... like, she did not die? Like, like, so O.M.G.

Attempt at sounding really, really hip and modern talk.

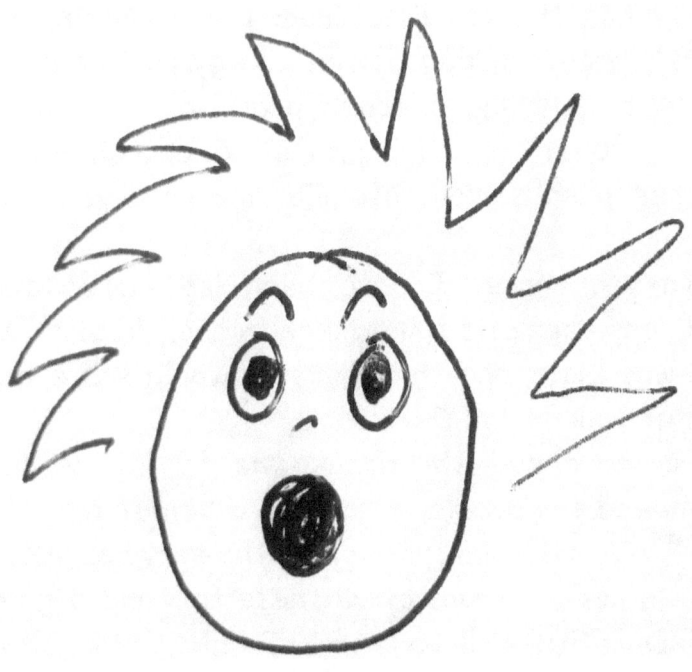

Chapter 22 - Brother Bob

I have never been much of a big church goer. Kinda lazy in the mornings. Kinda get my God from just waking up everyday. My farm has been my church. Actually, that is a literal statement now, because there is an adorable 7' x 9' Redneck pallet board chapel that we built in the summer of 2017, at the end of the property!

My church is also gazing up from my fields at a glorious mountain range, where fog frequently rolls in then lifts. The cover of this book was taken in my field! What the camera did not catch was my 3 miniature horses nibbling on my legs, then tipping the tripod over, while shooting! My church indeed! When the fog lifts from the mountain, it leaves an absolutely breath taking view of craggy rocks and evergreens. I 'spose too, having a foggy head so many mornings, and headaches to let lift, driving myself to church in the mornings sometimes wasn't even safe. For me or anyone else on the road!

In years past I have been led more toward open-minded, less dogmatic spiritual churches. Went to a Nazarene when I was little, and that minister would scare the hell into and out of you! HOLY CRAPOLA!

Having a dad who drank, the few times he and mom would attend for special occasions, often at the end was the: REPENT YOU SINNER portion of the service. Aka, git yer lil butt down here in front of all these folk and dag nabbit take the LORD JESUS CHRIST AS YER PERSONAL SAVIOR AND

YOU WILL BE ALL FINE AND DANDY IN HEAVEN WHEN YOU DIE! Me sitting there with my eyes big as saucers. The next scene, my dad would head to the alter and suddenly be the subject of prayer, and the preacher doin' his evangelistic thingy and dad crying. Well, this did nothin' more than make our family embarrassed. The drink is strong. When the soul is weak, Jesus has to work over-time. But heck, he liked wine too!

So I got a nasty taste in my mouth for hell, fire and damnation and... segregation! YES. Boy, howdy, did that ol' boy love to tell us all about DISCERNMENT. You must DISCERN or judge your brother and sister to be sure they are not toting the devil around in their skin.

Who needs brain injury, with crap like that coming from a holy building! Talk about FOG in belief systems! Stuff like: You know, cuz here, we believers, we are saved. And if you don't understand someone else's faith or lack of - they MUST be the devil! Hmmpf. (Learned that one from EOR Whinnie the pooh's pal). Another profound expression from my Grampa, who had horses that fit my thoughts on the private club. If he did not agree, he would pretend to sneeze and say "bull shit." I loved that. I must admit, I have done that a time or two in life.

When it comes to individuals learning about life, and when folks declare they have the one and only truth - and the rest of us are, well, heathen-hell-bounds, (unless they can earn brownie points by saving our souls with their belief system), my lil' farm mentality says that with nearly 8 billion people inhabiting this planet, and earth being a spec of dust in the big cosmos – that one group's belief about life and God, probably is just that. One belief. I would never "bull shit" sneeze to someone who merely said they are on a path. Respecting others. Sharing what they have learned so far. Only those that use it as power. Might cause me to sneeze.

Sayin' all this, stickin' my toes back in church-ish energy has been done with DISCERNMENT all right... to make SURE I did NOT feel judged walkin' in. To see if I had to believe how THEY believed or if I really could just show up for the coffee and cookies afterward, and maybe get a little gentle soul food too. Weeee!

Well, in my own search, not into clubs and exclusive at all, I found the more enlightened, new thoughtish open door church more fitting. I loved the word UNITY. I loved the word SPIRITUAL. SPIRIT. Shoot even that word, SPIRIT, has some ooobie dooobie vibes in some churches, like floppin on the floor and speakin a new language.

To me, it simply means: we are spiritual beings in human suits. We are light, if you will, energy for sure, clothed in flesh with these incredible brains that run the whole show. Talk about a generous Creator!

To see beautiful brains, all born as tiny babies, turn so full of hatred through generations and to turn spirits getting the human experience - against spirits, has broken my heart over and over. Even as a little girl. I just could not understand aggressive, in-your-face, self-righteous behavior.

I had to set up the stage for this chapter to tell you a game changer moment for me. I finally got my lazy, foggy brain and fanny to attend a Unity church service. There, I met an incredible man that really lit my soul up... named Brother Bob. He traveled the world as a motivational speaker and author, and has had the most jaw-dropping stories of finding self-worth and compassion - and his depth of spirituality. He had recently become the minister for that church. They had been without a preacher for a long time. Brother Bob - fit our Northwest Bellingham, Washington energy perfectly.

Talking to some of the congregation, I heard that with Brother Bob's talks, he had taken them much wider in thinking than it had gone before. Really teaching about connectedness, communicating and practicing the stuff he shared. About busting through FEAR and so on. I attended a few services and truly was moved.

When I learned that Brother Bob offered counseling at the church, I asked for an appointment. Something told me, we would connect much deeper than just spiritual talk. Our journeys. But not sure what that would mean til I showed up. Something I normally do not do, was I brought my guitar. It is generally not comfortable for me to sit face to face with a person to share a new song. But I felt strongly that I had 2 songs to share. Not being too comfy with counseling, as it were, I wasn't even sure how clear I could keep my brain. Perhaps I brought my guitar case along as my ol' friend. A grounding rod for Laurie.

Brother Bob was welcoming. Immediately we launched into similar areas we shared. Both had had numerous concussions and the long journey and struggles back. Both married 3 times. Both been in the music/entertainment world. Both been misunderstood by being in the public eye. Both knew abuse. Both knew depression and lack of self worth and the climb like hell, to get a little essence of heaven here on earth. WOW.

Nearing the end of our visit, Brother Bob asked me something. He asked, "How have the concussions served you?" I had not thought about them exactly as a service mode, but quickly came back with a couple things.

1. I saw that when we are mindful, we are more present. For me, when I was out to lunch too far ahead or thinking too far in the past, I would bonk my head. Not that those bonks brought me all that present. Heck no, instead, spaced out and foggy. But, made me ask myself, "where is your head? What are you doing?"

2. I noticed my fear level was lower and felt a bit more

courageous to do things. Carefully, and still afraid of committing to too much, due to souvenir things like migraines and bad balance. But still felt a little gutsier.

3.   I didn't care as much what others thought. THAT was huge.

4.   What we think about. Words. Patterns. How powerful they are. And how we seem to waste so much time on negative thought patterns and over-thinking things. Also, that while I already was a heart-centered person, this whole concussion stuff really opened my heart.

Listing these things was nice, until he asked me if I was done? I stalled out. Was I done hitting my head. 19 hits (at the time) and 1 bouncy truck shake up... was I done?   With the concussion experience? I said, "YUP!"

We talked about my farm. Organic farming. Helping grow for the food banks and the good life I had there.

Another big topic was about ever loving again. Brother Bob's passion to say "Love and love again. Get hurt. Heal. Love again!" That one was a tough subject. But deep in my core, I know he is right.

Before our time was up, I grabbed my guitar, and without much nervousness, I sang two songs to Brother Bob. SPIRIT PLAYING HUMAN and told him this is my biggest dream to record a healing music CD with this title, and a second meditative song called GO WITHIN.

Brother Bob grinned his gracious, handsome, loving grin and suggested I set a one year goal. That in a year, I would be performing my music and doing something I had never dreamed of. He lovingly reminded me, that "many can farm" but not everyone was gifted with my ability to sing and write songs. Then, he told me: it was TIME.

Almost a year to the day, I found myself asked up on the stage at the church, to tell folks that we were holding a big food drive at the church, due to a song I had written called: WHO WILL FEED THE HUNGRY. And about a CD called the Garden of my Soul that I had just released to raise money and awareness for Seattle's Northwest Harvest.

Brother Bob saw in me, something I had either forgotten or put on a shelf to be brought out when I was ready. I will never forget that special conversation that day, and the fact that my daughter and I sang SPIRIT PLAYING HUMAN for its first debut, and received a standing ovation.

Sometimes, we can be the FOG LIFTER for another person. Just a little encouragement. Being a good listener. Having compassion for their pain. Their journey. Not judging or telling them what to do. But identifying with them because we each know pain. Have been there. Maybe not the same injury. But pain and healing is pain and healing. Time and love are the greatest medicines.

Brother Bob was a fog lifter for me. He held up a loving mirror that said, "You will be okay, sister. YES you really have been through a lot. A LOT! But that is what makes our stories authentic."

Yes it takes mountains of courage, yes it is hard, yes it can be very dark, try to believe that your experience expands you. You may feel very limited right now. I have. I still do at times. I cannot say for sure if I am done hitting my head. Hells bells, I am a farmer. But, the core of my learning says, "Kiddo, take these things, and somehow grow deeper, stronger, more knowing and expand. Even if you have days you cannot stand up and walk straight or remember words to songs YOU have written, don't give up. Reach out. Help someone else."

With all my heart, *Thank you* beyond these words, Brother Bob. I know a couple counselors and neurologists that could learn a thing or two from you! I love you.
Love your little soul sissy, Laurie

Song lyrics: When the fog lifts

In groovy cool minor chords:

WHEN THE FOG LIFTS
verse 1:
I'll bet we've all – had times – in our lives
when the fog just got too thick.
To know an answer – or see through the other side
time was the measuring stick -
we're forced to - slow down - on the road we're on
so we won't crash or collide.
It's amazing – what can happen
if we take the time...

CHORUS
WHEN THE FOG LIFTS AND THE SUN COMES OUT
THE RAYS OF LIGHT – SHININ' ALL ABOUT
THERE - THE ANSWERS WAIT FOR US TO SEE.
WE CANNOT SEE A RAINBOW - IF THERE IS NO RAIN,
LESSONS MAY NOT FEEL GOOD - ENDURING SO MUCH
PAIN
BUT IT'S IN THOSE LESSONS – THAT WE CAN KNOW
THE GIFT...
WHEN THE FOG LIFTS... WHEN THE FOG LIFTS.

Verse 2

One might think they – have life all figured out.

Nothin' can stop the path their on.
Fog may roll in – road disappearin'
wonderin' if tomorrow – will even come?
Straining to see – so exhausting,
finally – taking deep breaths of faith
letting go and letting God
replacing fog with love's grace.

CHORUS

WHEN THE FOG LIFTS AND THE SUN COMES OUT
THE RAYS OF LIGHT – SHININ' ALL ABOUT
THERE - THE ANSWERS WAIT FOR US TO SEE.
WE CANNOT SEE A RAINBOW - IF THERE IS NO RAIN,
LESSONS MAY NOT FEEL GOOD - ENDURING SO MUCH
PAIN
BUT IT'S IN THOSE LESSONS - THAT WE CAN KNOW
THE GIFT...
WHEN THE FOG LIFTS... WHEN THE FOG LIFTS.

Words & music by Laurie Lee Lewis,
Copyright 2012-Lewis BMI

Chapter 23 - Local Love Light Librarians

I live in a very tiny, blink-and-you'll-miss-it pass through teeny town. Literally one small cool landmark store full of organic foods and imported cheese has just closed its doors after almost 50 years. The family has owned the store since I was in grade school. My dad and I went to the same grade school, my folks, daughter and I all graduated from the same high school.

There is good and there is bad to living in the same town folks saw you as a freckle-faced, pig-tailed lil gal riding your pony.   History. My music, modeling, humanitarian endeavors have been in the news, radio, television... and folks have had impressions of the Laurie who recorded a CD. Or helped build a neighbor a house, or raised money for animals or hungry people. Or saw my cds in stores, or knew I toured in the 90s' or saw me singing in a band.

All these things are tiny slivers of a person. The good is - if they know you long enough, a few may know when you go through the foggy stuff. The divorce. The moves. The concussions. But, then if you surface again, as I have, and suddenly doing music again, they forget you have had any injuries. (So do I) ... but a few, remember. When people only want to remember you as the singer or model, it is much harder to be out in public. There is one constant place that has never mattered what condition I was in, where I have always been greeted kindly. The library.

I want to take a couple seconds here to share an

experience with our local librarians. I am not a big reader but have enjoyed borrowing DVDs to watch at home. I am almost always greeted by 3 or 4 regular faces. "Hi Laurie, how are you doing?" Anyone of them will ask as I walk through the doors, probably in my farm boots, hat, bibs, trying not to drag in dirt. Goodness knows the many faces that they have seen by Laurie Lee Lewis, in my post-concussion, post-dad dying, humanitarian, caregiver burnout and/or just keeping up with life, *quick* library stops.

Through my ordeals, many times I could not stay in the library very long. The books and busy of the shelves would mess with my eyes. The lights. The chance of running into someone and having to carry on a conversation could be over-whelming. I do very well, now! But never take it for granted!

On one visit I was touched so deeply by such a kindness that comes from librarians. Truly wanting to help you. Our gals are wonderful. Soft spoken, asking about my farm and life. Sincerely engaging.

On one trip to the library, I was befuddled. A few days before, I had returned a stack of DVDs. But I got a notice that one, I had just returned the case, no DVD. Which isn't that unusual for me. They are use to finding a Ziploc bag with the disc, smiley face and an apology note. This time, I had gone in to ask if they received my Ziploc return. They had not. I was so confused and my mind was obsessing on remembering returning it. But a piece was missing.

As I shared this, one of the librarians who knows my story - graciously stepped up and said, "Well, look again, and if you can't find it, and you really think you returned it Laurie, we will take care of it so you won't have to pay for it." I think I saw a sweet wink. My heart went up in my throat.

I felt so lucky that these wonderful women worked here. A few days later, my dad found the DVD slipped under the seat of his car. Left there the day I took them to their doc appointments.

Another librarian knew that I had met a lovely man and was going to try again in the love department. Asked about that in one of my stop-ins.

Another knows how hard I worked to help my neighbor when he got in a chainsaw accident severing his arm 95% off. Who was flown to Seattle for surgery. While he was gone, care-taking his dogs and cat, we found that his home had burned from the inside, and he was living in this disaster for several years like a hermit. I mounted a large effort to improve his home.

With neighbors joining together, we did not remodel his old house, we built him a new one. It was a mammoth act of love. I even told the story at that library and we took up an offering that night with teary eyes thanking me for stepping up.

So as I left the library, I remembered back on how many times that it was all I could do just to drive that 5 miles to find a little movie and come home. I truly realized how I have always felt appreciated, walking in and seeing those love lights. Librarians rock! Local heroes of gentle, quiet and gracious kindness!

I imagine, if you are deep in the fog or you love someone in that state, these words are probably not the only ones you have read about regarding TBI (Traumatic Brain Injury) or concussion or concussions, brain injuries...

I will say the library has some very fine books about brain injury. The only thing I discovered was - that most of the ones I checked out, did not speak lamens words from inside the concussion. AS I said in the beginning of this book, I saw the technical, medical verbiage that I could not even pronounce. Or, injury but then they healed and told everyone else you will heal. But still, not the book that said: *While I MAY BE CHALLENGED WITH THIS FOREVER, I can still do* something with my life. I may always have trouble with certain environments, limitations, mini seizures if too tired or stressed. I don't know. Truth is, I might hit again. You might.

Since I did not find the book I was looking for, well, I wrote one! YUP YUP YUP. I declared, somehow, I would hold on, use this to help others.

Hey, hey, lookie there, you are reading it! Hot damn. Life is amazing! I kept my promise to my dad, to write this and share my story.

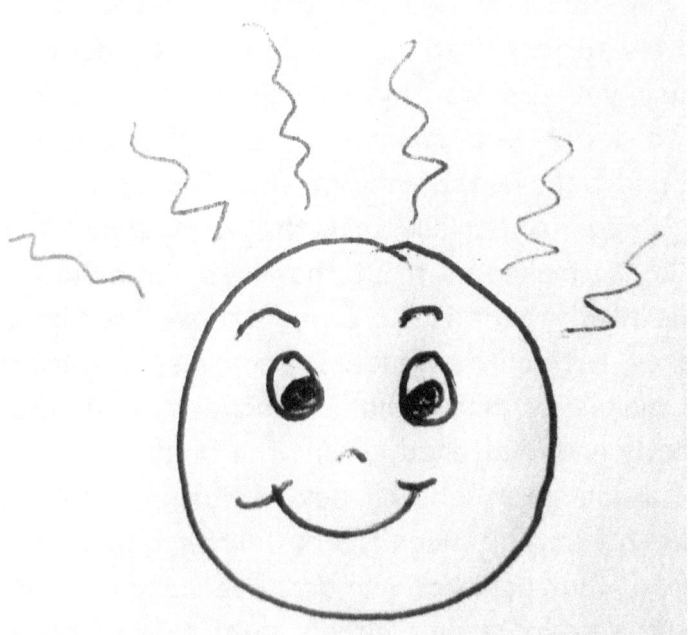

This I know for myself:

We have NOW and what comes in the next NOW. We can choose to dwell in the dark. The story. The injury. The pain. Or, we can choose to try to shift and look at some of the love lights in our lives. See blessings that we may never have seen before, that were right there - if we had not gotten injured.

Chapter 24 - TRUST

Boy howdy, this subject, TRUST - popping up in a brain injury book - is a ddd-doozy! As you probably have already read, you are putting your head and ass on the line when you step out to survive and thrive in this life. Especially when you are in the fog and try to just keep up. Trying to be productive. Trying to remember you are worthy. Trying to remember the fog is trying to teach you *something*. Oh, and the big one, too TRUST and believe that any of the "fog-as-a-teacher" ... can be a huge page in your soul growth. Whew-skies!

No one makes us trust that idea. Or believe it. No one makes us trust there is a creator of love that gave us life to experience, with all its wonders, beauties, with highs and lows. No one makes us trust that we have a brain that runs our entire body and if altered, alters the body. Scientists (those wonderful souls, in labs all day, devoting their lives to find out more about our magnificent human being stuff) ... have discovered what parts of our brain operate what parts of our body. Left side of brain controls right side of body. Wow. Hit on the right side of your head, brain flies over to the left side of your skull, so which side is screwed up? Well, it can be both sides of course. The side that took the blow and the side that receives the impact.

Your neurological symptoms may not reveal themselves immediately - because that is a whole lot of wiring to traumatize. Can you imagine dropping your lap top or PC brain. Turning it on and see if it crashed?

I decided to touch on TRUST because in my fog lifting and growing experiences, trust shows up EVERYWHERE. Or lack of it.

We have to TRUST a doctor or surgeon or MRI technician, providing the machine doesn't eat our brain while in the tube getting the MRI! And, of course, the radiologists who read our reports.

We have to TRUST when we hear or say: I LOVE YOU, that those words come from the heart, not some conditional state from the other person or your self - because of need. Loneliness. Desperation. Possessiveness. Or even just saying it habitually - without heart. Or someone you don't really know and they say goodbye to you with a "love ya" and you think to yourself, "huh?" Becoming patterned creatures rather than heart-based souls.

We have to have TRUST when we bring a child into this world, that no matter how we ended up getting there, believing this child is meant to be.

We have to have TRUST that when your brain is completely fine and dandy on a Monday, taking a little spin on a bicycle, horse, skates, skateboard, trampoline, or whatever... that Tuesday, we will wake up with the same brain. But for some of us, we don't. And then, a whole new level of TRUST has to enter in - as HOPE, that somehow we will glean from this, grow from this and be able to LIVE.

As I keep saying, I have no medical experience. Only the experience of a life - that put me right on the very edge of a cliff (once, literally) that showed me each of us exist here on earth, taking another breath by choosing to stay on the cliff. Not jump. Not give up. If someone pushes us, well shoot, probably the story is over... unless of course YOU are one of those unbelievable survivors that actually fell off the cliff and reading this - for some hope. If you are, dang, I want to read YOUR book!

TRUST enters in - when we choose to love again, after brutal pain that wounds the heart deeply. TRUST that you can *trust again*, if you were abused at any time of your life. TRUST appears when you look in a mirror for weeks, months, or longer and cannot see yourself or even remember what you are doing here. Some seed of trust that you will reappear. YOU will come back. You will heal. You may be different than you were before that ride, walk, drive but YOUR life is here for a purpose. And maybe, up til now, you have focused primarily on pleasing - YOU? Suddenly your new life experience becomes about service to others. Time for them to TRUST you!

I am so grateful at this point, that I can remember so much. I know at any given moment our memories can be taken away.   You see it with Dementia/Alzheimers.   You wonder where they went? Shadows of their former selves.

What makes us wake up with even the smallest TRUST? Is it faith? That God has created this life right on track and going to use you somehow to inspire others? What if you don't believe in God? Or GOOD? As I mentioned earlier. What if you have lived your life in *FEAR OF GOD. FEAR OF GOOD.* Then how in the heck, do we get back to saying: WHEN THE FOG LIFTS... I will rise up... I will use this for the HIGHEST GOOD?

I remember it being a huge achievement to be able to bend over and put on my shoes without falling over. To go to a movie theater and not have to leave because of the motion and volume.

I remember on a New Year's eve, going down to the local community hall and dancing without vertigo or falling. Huge night for this brain. The littlest things. Remembering songs to sing. Seeing myself for the first time in months in a mirror and saying, "I know you."   To be able to drive myself and my elderly parents to doctor appointments or Sunday outings. To grocery shop. And the list goes on. TRUST that I would somehow get better then I was - gave me HOPE.

So I 'spose, if you lined these words all up, you could do your own order.

Is it trust, hope, faith?

Is it faith, hope, trust?

Is it hope, faith, trust?

Is it hope, trust, faith?

Not important, just kind of a riddle-type fun. To mess with us. No matter what order, is it possible in your fog, that one of those variations of 3 words hopefully will let you experience the ultimate love: Unconditional love!

Believe me, when you scramble those eggs upstairs and people suddenly are around a different version of you, all kinds of stuff surfaces! Friends, much like if you quit drinking, may not want to be around you, or they will surprise you and want to be close, to let you know they care. People get scared of altered brains.

Recently, I was talking to a friend who told me that whenever she sees someone in a wheel chair or walker, she intentionally makes eye contact and somehow tries to get the message across that she sees them, and cares. Then will ask if they are having a good day. Some kind effort to show them she does not fear their limitation. She doesn't think they are invisible or contagious. She remembers that at any moment, the shoes could switch and it could be her. And how lovely it would be, if she was struggling - to get through a day, through a doorway, whatever it may be, that some nice person, smiled, and saw her. Helped her. Wished her a lovely day. That really rocked it for me. Shifted me, actually.

TRUST that you are not alone. Someone, somewhere, will arrive on your path, if needed, to help you... You may have to lower your own pride. Let someone in. Let someone help. Especially, if up til now, like me, you had a *I WILL DO IT*

MYSELF mentality. Afraid to bother another person. Laurie, can you read that last line that your fingers just typed!

Or you think you could do it best. Oh gosh, there is so much to this letting down the guard, when the fog lifts, to find out we need each other. And have to learn to TRUST.

I trust that I can trust you?
As I lay my defenses on the ground.
That you will let me tell my truth
Not judge or knock me down.

I trust that you can trust me.
In what you need to say.
That I will be there for you.
Anytime, any day.
LLL

Chapter 25 - Fog and choices

This book would certainly not be authentic comin' from this brain if I did not write a time or two IN the actual fog. I think I have done that. Mostly though, I have said in the previous chapters that *time* and *hope* have been the best medicines. I will stick to that til my last breath. Because there have been many times I thought I could not possibly wake up in the morning with so much pressure in my brain all night, and that surely this was the big one that would kill me.

Now that is a dag gum dramatic statement, but in the LONG times, LONG days, LONG nights, sure, those thoughts were there. So, rather than dwell in those windows, I told myself something pretty important. This subject is a tough one. You may start reading and not be ready to read it. I understand. I wasn't going to write it.

Today, I am in the fog. Yes, spell check has asked, "huh?" a few times. Okay more than a few. But, I am determined to write what is in my head and heart NOW.

In the world, on the news, in our families, neighborhoods, our jobs and communities, we have incoming information. What might start as a gentle talk with a neighbor, might lead into conflict talk. Opinions of another. To some degree, if it is illegal actions taking place next door, like shooting, labs, drug sales, and the list goes on, that is a tough one. I believe you have the right - to expose them, stop them, before someone gets hurt. Tricky part is, you also endanger yourself.

On the news, that one is even trickier. You cannot

change the news. It is in a little box, that takes a power switch. Behind the box is producers, an anchor, words read from a paper that were written perfectly to be NEWS. Unless it is live of course.   Most of us know that politics and religion divide lives, families, states, countries!   Our civilization just isn't advanced as a whole yet, to see the bigger picture of how we become puppets on strings. Told what to believe. Once we do wake up to this, then it is choice.

So we choose.   Every day, we choose, what we let be our reality. If the power goes out and you have no lights, you light a candle. If the water isn't on, YOU IS IN BIG TROUBLE if you have to poop! Okay, the farm chick had to throw in a funny.   But other people's thoughts and opinions, are just that. THEIRS!

So many would never imagine not having their brain working in full operation. Others just suck up coffee. Pop. Red Bull. Drugs. Cocaine. Whatever gets them ramped to get through and power on, another day.   So hard to include my friend, Mr. Coffee.

We are like herbs.   HUH? You say.   When cooking, we can make the most incredible dishes. Do everything right. But then, what was suppose to be, Rosemary, was, Thyme.   Or Ginger was garlic. Suddenly a perfect dish changed direction in flavors. Well, depending on your culinary abilities and creativity, you either scratch the dish or shift it into something different.

Weird analogy, but I think that is sometimes how I feel when I wake up each morning. Anything can happen. Totally different than what I thought.   Someone might be having a really bad day and decide it would be less bad if they dumped it on me.   Or the news on my computer/TV is splattered with sex scandals, President updates, and so on, not one of them can I change.

The only thing I can do – is change the channel. Power

off. Not listen. Decide to shift the spice into something good by coming back to Mr. or Ms. Bad-day dumper and say, "YAH, but we are still alive. Another day with this beautiful GIFT called life."   They may shrug. But ya know what? Down the road, from their foggy morning to perhaps clear skies, someone will come to them in a bad way, and they, who's to say, might just use your words! Chain reaction.

You chose not to let the world around you win. Not let the garlic ruin what was suppose to be ginger. Okay, if you were making molasses-ginger cookies, this principle is just NOT gonna work. You can try it, but... eeew!

I just want to be a reminding voice. Other people also have fog. They may or may not be as humble and cool as you on any given day.   They might want to blame somebody.   I remember back in the day, how some of my pals would blame the world for their HANG-OVER!   Ha! We do not know what is going on in another person's life. Much like driving. Did they just lose their job, loved one, medical news and beyond? Fog?

For the absolute ones that you just know are programmed and need to bitch - you are not responsible for their life. Never were, never are.   You ARE responsible for your own.   So when you wake up in a fog, as I am today, I have to remember a few things:

I have not hit for some time. I am okay. Truth is, I stayed up late. Ate something sugary before I went to sleep, messing with my blood sugars in the morning. I have not had enough water, so my brain is probably dehydrated. Owning some of my actions and knowing what I can do to help. Take a nap. Drink water. Get some fresh air. Stay off the phone if I can. Type for only a few minutes at a time and know that this will lift.

Part of what I apparently feel to share here is that we choose all day long - not maybe who or what comes in, but what we do with it. Jump on the band wagon and get angry,

175

sayin "yah" when a post like of a little dog is humpin' a stuffed Trump doll on Facebook appears in front of you - with a beyond-low opinion tagged to it and a million likes! Forgetting one key thing: us, in a mirror. Anger/hate feeds anger/hate.

Ten years from now, this will not make any sense. So why do we buy into opinions so easily. We use to call this bad manners, in grade school. We got sent to the corner. Time out. Johnny had to say he was sorry to Jimmy. But we grow up and become the sum total of everyone else's opinions, fears, and thoughts - if we aren't careful. If don't wake up to our own thoughts, thus we become puppets. Even if it takes a clobber to the computer on our shoulders, or in my case, many. It sometimes has felt like the universe has had to keep me in the fog, so I would go deeper into my soul, rather than "out there".

I find this all pretty amazing. With no agenda, as my foggy head receives these words, and fingers try to type them, I have no idea what is coming out next. So I guess the message to you is: PAY ATTENTION to incoming energy, and opinions!

After one hit, I went off of Facebook for over a year. Could not look at a computer screen for a long time. So these things that we assume are our lives. Our MUST HAVES to exist, well, we created. We bought into it. In fact, all the fear of global warming and earth tipping on its axis and terrorists and, and, and... all the things that are out there to fuel our fears. If we did not have news, we would live day to day. Like remote villages do today.

If the earth tipped, mountains fell, well we would know, a minute before, but not hold fear every day of: WHAT IF. I know folk can argue this, but I would much rather spend the time trying to be a healthier, happy person, than worry. Fear lowers our immune systems. Worry creates distraction from being present, and that, is when accidents happen.   Learning to be good to yourself and others, that is when blessings happen.

Part two of this seems to want to come out now -

Trust me, I am not pretending I am some guru channeling great fog-lifting information here. I am just rolling with it! I will go somewhere valuable or I will erase it! I promise. Although I must say, I *have* been known to dress up as nutty Psychic Suzie, telling fortunes, using fortune cookies!

When Y2K was about to shift from 1999 to 2000 the world really was worried what was going to happen with our world-based computers.   Everything. Dams, traffic lights, medical/hospitals, anything and everything is dependent on a computer or computer chip. There was a lot of scrambling in Microsoft world. 2000 arrived, we were okay.

The folks that were really concerned, cleaned out stores with supplies, felt the end-times, fear of desperation and what could happen.   One event like that - really woke some people up. Wondering if things like jets could suddenly come crashing down on our heads due to no computer. Lost ships. Trains that would not stop, and so on. This is a far-out way to get to this: We came through it. Perhaps some thought about end times. Others, as I said, bought up supplies. We are still here.   In light of natural disasters, being self-sufficient, instead of totally dependent on available things – is indeed very wise. *Very* wise. It reminds us of the big picture.

There is another picture.

As you read this, perhaps you live at home with family. Perhaps you have your own family. Or the caregiver. So often, we live like we will live forever, so the joke of the "round toit" means eventually I will get to it.

When you are healing - you cannot do it all. You will make yourself miserable if you try. But there is one thing I have been thinking about a lot and, yes, I have put it off too, but starting to change that. To get a notebook. To write down or have someone write down, not a journal as much as your wishes if you should die. I had huge talks with my 80's parents knowing time was ticking.

At first they did not want to even discuss the idea of dying. Of course. But one day, I said to mom, real love, isn't just loving another person. It is loving them so much that YOU take the time to say what you want if you die. A few wishes like: do you want to be cremated or a casket. Donated to science? Big/little service? What songs? Any favorite poems or writings? Favorite photos?

Think about it. You have made it this far without dying. Me too. Bravo us! Some are so attached to things they own, this idea of the end is terrifying. To me, I have a lot of stuff. Crap. CDs stuffed in closets. Animals. And thoughts. Well, less thoughts, as I type them out here! Lol!

The question and conversation I had with my mom to help her help me, was, "I think love should include that I do not have to make those BIG choices when you die, when you are here, right now. You could do that for or with me!" That is self-less love. Instead of: "No way man, I am not talking about that stuff, deal with it when I die and all my stuff."

But think about it, these people, sometimes just one or two key people will suddenly lose their loved one. Perhaps they will be completely exhausted from the loss and, maybe the journey to the final day. Especially caregivers. So now you have a child, spouse, parent or friend that has to create a memorial. Then deal with bills, death certificates, home, stuff – let alone, try to make room for grief!

Wow, even as I type this, I am thinking about all my

crap and what my poor daughter will have to unload.   So maybe not just listing my wishes and instructions, but start unloading some of the crap now! The latest books, shows, and posts are all about the fact that stuff, believe it or not, doesn't make our lives bigger. Just more cluttered.

So depending on where these words find you – if you simply can pick up a small tablet, something that if you have a Will, you can have it attached to, or just written in, and tell someone "my last wishes."   What will happen by doing this, is if your brain can go to these areas (depends on the state of mind, literally) the reflection of YOU being given this life in all its facets, will come forward.

Now if this stresses you, reading this, just take it as a loving hug from me. I had no intention of bringing you more stress.   My soul just felt it necessary to bring this information to this part of the book. YOU do not need more stress or pressure if you are healing.

Even if it is freaky weird to talk about, I had to do it in joking form at some points with my daughter, but more serious at other times.   I think in some ways, she was relieved.   I can only imagine, losing mom and then the nightmare of dealing with mom's trail and world.

Having no idea what your world is like, maybe you already have your act together, and these words are nothing new. If so, wow, kudos to yudos!

Today's foggy brain tells me that I delivered the messages here.

Thanks for traveling through this part with me.

I choose to love
I choose to live -
I choose to be
the love I give.

I choose to believe
that life is a gift -
when I learn and grow
I see the fog lift.

LLL

Chapter 26 -
What I have learned about me?

Have you ever asked this question? *What have I learned about me?* It is a lil' toughy, if your pride is still ruling your soul. Filling your ego with rightness. If not, this question is *amazing*. A reflection of who are you now.

I think of all the people in my life, past and present. The loves that have come and gone. The tears poured and laughter laughed. Mistakes that might look differently if we suddenly see the "aha" that show us: *if that would not have happened that way, I would not have met that person or gone in that place.* Sometimes, this can really fun to look at.

Now to some, if you are in a rough state right now, you may be looking back, thinking: "Skitskies, if only I would NOT have done this or that, or stayed home, wore a helmet, said I was sorry, or I love you - or did not drink, slowed down and the list goes on and on, right? Guilt, remorse, loss. All fog.

When you wake up to this FOG, and your computer hard drive has crashed (this includes mental break downs here) and all you see if NOTHIN' - impossible, too thick... *again*, we have to decide inside ourselves (because only *we* can) *which* direction will we take this foggy experience. Power up to say, what can I learn from this, right now? A surrender to what we thought life would be, and open to use what is - NOW.

If you are smack in the middle of an angry divorce or tanked on pain medications daily, that's a powerful FOG. OR locked in your house on your computer or phone all day on social media or playing video games, well, guess what? That too, a powerful FOG. Especially if you feel something is missing in your life.

Here is another FOG: Any excess of what I call: the Laurieism, country-fied "g-less" word list. As we wonder why our lives are so full of FOG: It's fun to say, but packs a punch, especially if you look at yourself right now, and some of these words might resonate with your "currant life." Brain-injured or not! Ready?

Smokin', tokin', blamin', chewin',
snortin', shootin', cheatin', screwin',
gossipin' gorgin', textin', drinkin'
stealin', fightin', hatin'-thinkin'!

Want to know what is even more irritating than this list? Now say them all with the G back on each word. Really enunciate! DANG! Your face gets really tired of these words quickly! Can you imagine what your body, mind and spirit feel, on a cellular level? Talk about FOG! I could pert near end this book right now. 'Nuff said. But I won't. Cuz I am full of it!

Remember, I am no scholarly shrink, brainyologist, or counselor. I am a brain that has sustained bumps, thumps and dumps and just using it to channel this stuff! I don't mean: DON'T LIVE! Or even stop all that stuff, I just ask, WHAT IS FOGGING UP OUR LIFE? It might not be an injury. It might be OUR choices! And, the excuses about OUR choices.

Now, the missing "g" in livin', lovin', laughin', and learnin' - well, that is totally different. Awesome, abundant, astonishing and amazing! Sorry, my fingers have taken over and are on a roll here.

Ya see, I did not write this book just to say, "Ooopsie, I smacked my noggin' 20 times. Pity please! Certainly not "POOR ME." That one would make me puke! It is about: LIFE HAPPENS. And, if you believe in any form of: there is a REASON WHY IT HAPPENS, then you take these big ffffoggies - and start asking for it to reveal something. But if you believe that life is random, yer born, live, die and life sucks, you are a total victim, you are floating randomly through life until it comes to an end well, my lil' stories probably will go right over head. Not to your heart.

You are no worse off than before you read these words. Honestly. No damage. But if you read them, and some little whisper of *possibility* speaks to you, sayin' that you are right where you are suppose to be RIGHT NOW, I swear (and I do, sometimes) that *THAT* is when shift begins. *THAT* is when Fog starts to lift on our lives, and when you ask the question: "What have I learned about me?" Ooooh doggies. Giddy-up! Yahoosky! Becoming your own best friend - instead of worst enemy, is the answer to a lot of fog.

I have learned many things that have helped me pull through - to write this book. I have learned that since I was a little girl, I did not really trust. Particularly men. But have had many men in my life. As dear friends, sweeties, obsessed jealous and scary men, brainy men, common sense men. Forgiving men. Unforgiving men. And for much of my life, ironically, it was usually easier for me to talk to men, then women. I 'spose I have developed my masculine side enough, to totin' around cordless drills and tools, that I could relate better to the masculine side.

The women I have been closest to have been a mix. Some, very feminine. The nails, the hands, the run, the gestures - while others, like me, not so feminine. But to most of them, I suppose they looked at me and might shake their heads, at my grubby work attire and dirty face and fingernails. (At least during farm season.) I can scrub up.

I am not fearless. Plenty scares me. Bumps in the night make my heart race. Facing someone to set something straight has terrified me. I hate fighting. I hate disagreeing. Mostly because I have memories of that getting really mis-understood, not followed through with forgiveness, grudges made, and just never seen it done lovingly. Once you have been picked up by your throat, by a very out-of-control man, or screamed on til you faint, some things stand out that you just never want to re-create. Even when you are safe. Deep memories. Trust can feel like a distant word.

So my nature has been, even though with the total of my 3 marriages, 26 years worth, I still felt like a lone ranger often. Sharing a life. A house. A bed. The bills. Whatever. But when it came down to getting things done, in my brain, I often did not ask for help. I would just jump in and do it myself. Well, I still do.

This is hard for me to admit. But I asked the question. So I should answer it.   Was it that I really thought my partner could not do it as well as me? Or was there a sense that if I asked, either they would say okay, and I would wait and wait, or I would hear 20 ways to do it?   I have a mind that sees and does. Maybe not right, but I really dislike verbal work that may or may not result in action. Got my daddy's blood. Git'r done or go home! This can be a double-edged sword. Especially when you are capable, mostly. Until you get injured.

So, if you sit with me, and tell me: I'm a GONNA DO THIS AND I'm a gonna do THAT... but I look and see that you are one who never leaves your couch, computer chair, the television or whatever - my knees will probably get tappin'. I will want MY TIME on this earth back, rather than sit and listen to you and all your dreams. I am so sorry. Really. Different strokes for different folks. Remember, part of lifting fog is asking what you have learned about yourself, so far?

By the way, the above knee tappin'... if I have done this to you, I apologize. But I am a git'r done, shit or get-off- depot woman. That does not make me a good woman. It is just what kind of farmer, singer, songwriter, producer and help others - woman, I am. It gets things done. Food grown.

I 'spose I would call myself a smidgin' IMPATIENT. Grin. Since hitting my head so many times in 10 years, having to recover 6 months from a full blown hysterectomy, etc., I feel the time clock ticking. Like I do not want to sit and watch it go by. Hells bells, I had to already live that way with *chunks of time*, in deep fog, while healing, not barely do anything. I was stuck. So maybe I am making up for that time.

The big message here is: LIVE! As I think I have said already, thousands of words ago, how much I love the line from: MY FAIR LADY, as Audrey Hepburn watches the horse races. She is trying to be a proper lady all prettied up in a perfect dress and hat. With her strong Cockney accent right under her refined one - you see her watching. The horses are coming around the track. Audrey's gorgeous eyes widen and you hear her say: (properly at first) "Come on Dover, Come on Dover (Dover is the horse she bet on) and then... busts into her old accent yellin' loudly: "COME ON, DOVA, MOVE YOUR BLOOMIN' ASS!" (auss.) Shocking everyone. Stellar moment! I am an Eliza Doolittle. It makes perfect sense. After all, my birth last name is: Little!

I have been known to finally blow and say: "MOVE YOUR BLOOMIN'ASS or MOVE OUT." Essentially saying: NO FREE LUNCH. DO YOUR PART. YOU ARE NOT A VICTIM.
So again, I ask, "What have I learned about me?" hehehe

Well, if we look at what others say, through the years, hmmm, that one is tricky because they only see you from their perspective. But I have heard many things, and certainly made me double-take and ask myself: IS THIS YOU? Are they right? Do they know me more than I know me? Especially, when someone hears a new song, that I just finished and they want to change it. Or see a photo of me, and wish I did something different. Or, read this book, and focus on the enditing instead of the message.   We live in our brain.

Deciding if something is good enough. Instead of just being present to the blessing, we are scanning with opinions. I am trying to change that, in me.

What what do others say about me. Hmm, let's see, over the years... to name a few: Self-righteous, Devil-filled, ambitious, work-a-holic, narcissistic, self-absorbed, self-less, generous, kind, nice person, earth angel, selfish, heart-breaker, impatient, very patient, gentle, drama queen (I love that one), home wrecker, gutsy, survivor, honest, liar, talented, poor-me, unbelievable, hard worker, good friend, artist, spiritual, friendly, quiet, a trooper, inspiring.

I am sure there is at least 100 more words or "descriptions" that have been said. Partially when you chase dreams, achieve some of them, are in the public eye, or willing to be outspoken when it is needed, people are quick to assess and judge. Plenty of critics out there.

So then, then comes the question again,
"What have I learned about me?"

Well, when you start as a very shy little girl, who did not even look in the mirror. If someone said, "You are pretty" would shrug curled shoulders so as not to accept the compliment and appear self-righteous. Or that little girl heard: "SHOW OFF and STUPID" and you believed them. How can you not believe them, if you are a tender-heart?

So then that little girl travels life with these damn words haunting you. Even with achievements. You cannot shake them. *Worthiness* is so fragile, and gets lost so easily. If worthiness was our first message from birth and deeply ingrained in our DNA, of life-affirming tools, we would not have such a screwed up world. Psychotherapists would not have a job. But... most of us seem to have to learn this *little by little*. To be brave enough to lift fog and then, Own it and

LIVE our lives fully! By choice!

In reality: Most of us want that one person, who wounded you, to walk up some day and say "I am sorry. I admire you. You did good. Good job." *Anything* to shift the balance of why we do what we do. Truth is, once we realize this may or may never happen from that person, we have to shift. We have to decide they do not own our power. We do. We choose to forgive, learn-from, let go, or hold on. I blamed for years. Not consciously, but I did. When I finally looked at the worst memories, really looked, knowing I may not ever get an apology, I realized that apology and love will come from somewhere else, if I let go.

This does NOT mean that you cower down and not stand up for yourself. Hell and heavens - NO! I finally *did* stand up for myself. It took years. Not to everyone who hurt me, but to a couple deep ones. It HAD to happen. It was not until I got to truly speak for my beloved, yes, *beloved* self, (which was an exhausting) finally to say, "I DON'T CARE ANYMORE WHAT YOU THINK, *or even if you don't* LOVE ME!" WOW!

I realized that I would gladly protect someone - that I love. I'd give my life. WHY then, would I not do that for myself? What is that? When we truly love and respect ourselves, and believe we are worthy of a beautiful life... eventually we need to stand up and declare our worthiness.

I feel deep down inside - that I hurt myself over and over because in there, somewhere, my little being was trying to scream at me, "YOU do not feel worthy. So work your ass off, and even if you hurt yourself, so what." Weird huh?

Why did it take me 10 years of head injuries, in and out of the fog, and all the years before? Well, some of us just have thick heads! Well, not so thick, or I would not have had concussions with MRIs showing scars everywhere.

Somewhere in this life, when we ask who we are, what we have learned, we might ask the words that I wrote in my song, MIRROR:, inspired by the late, Louise Hay's phenomenal spiritual teachings:

"Somewhere, somehow, we might get the message
that we are not worthy,
to receive love, and deserve love
Looking in the mirror, I have to see me.

Wanting to be whole,
wanting to be healed,
Wanting to know love and set myself free...
so my new life an MIRROR me."
Louise, if you and Wayne Dyer can hear me, THANK YOU!

Being willing to look at ourselves, not others – ourselves, as we are now, either brain-injured and healing or one who loves the brain-injured and trying to understand more. Huge soul, fog-lifting stuff! Our belief systems can be a brain injury all by itself. Everything we were and are programmed to believe since childhood. So decoding all of that and coming out on the other side asking yourself: Is this really me or just how others perceive me, and I believed them? This lifts fog!"

We get an opportunity to look. Our brains might not even let us go there, during swelling, bleeding, healing... but at some point, there is a good chance that we will have a mirror of life held up to say, "How did I get here, and what have I learned about me? And, where do I go from here with this honest information?"

As you lift fog to honesty, ooof, that mirror, ya might want to break it, if you can even look in it. But it's worth it. If you find yourself in the FOG, and ask, "Do I have FEAR OF GOOD... good coming into my life? Do I deserve this? Finally to let yourself get ballsy and say, "YES I DO, damn straight! I was given this life for a reason. I AM WORTHY! I Am - as I

Am - now. To grow, heal, inspire!" **Unbelievable** things will happen. Fog will lift!

Little FYI here, if you happen to be one of the judgmental type, that have lists as above, of what you think about your relative, neighbor, friend - when you look in the mirror, when you *own* it, when you ask, WHAT HAVE I LEARNED ABOUT ME... When the fog lifts, you will see yourself, and that's when you shift. You will be amazed how fast all those judgmental words that quickly poured out about another... disappear. They have no value. No meaning. They are not important because you will have found and released - you.

You will know the value of what time you have left as YOU. And more than likely get living it. In whatever package you are in - NOW. This is pretty key stuff. It breaks patterns. It makes us uncomfortable but then, accountable. It makes us grateful that we get another breath, another chance to live.

We may still need help. If our brains are not working correctly and we are seriously depressed, we may need medicine. Vitamins. Herbs. Exercise. Counseling. Friends. Groups. Hobbies. It is letting the fog lift to be able to ask these things. It is okay to ask for help. We actually do need each other.

In my post-concussion hours, I had many "check out" windows of starring. Wasn't sure even how long I was gone. Sounds weird now. But I would come back and reality was hard to be in. Pile of dishes, clothes, yard, farm, bills, home-schooling stuff for my daughter. I would fill with anxiety and cry.

Writing this book now, no way, back then could I even type forward. But again, I prayed someday, so many hits, so many healings, so many blessings, nightmares and emotions that I would be able to share. To say, "If you are trapped in the fog, try to breathe in a little hope and trust that love will pull you through." The fog will lift. Hang in there. Please, FOR YOUR SOUL's JOURNEY... YOU are worthy, hang in there.

When the fog lifts, bravely, and lovingly ask, "What have I learned about me?"   Life is a gift. No matter what package it comes in. Open it. Be brave.   YOU are not a mistake. YOU are a GIFT. YOU are WORTHY! Start again.

On a lighter, nothing to do with the above, note here... I have been editing throughout spring, determined to finish this book. With farming season starting too, I have felt torn to sit and do this. But, wanted it released for Mother's day as a goal and a way to say THANK YOU to my mom, for all the years care-giving my dad. Just today, while editing ... I had an epiphany. (I think that is how ya spell it.) I realized, when ya pull weeds in your garden or flower beds, you reveal the beautiful plants.   I have been pulling weeds all month on this book to reveal something beautiful to share. You may still find a weed or many, but hopefully you can see the flowers and healthy produce too, in my words! The forest through the trees as Mr. Thoreau reminded us.

I am cool. I am not.
I get gas. I get snot.
Gross you out? I don't care.
We aren't here, to compare.
~
Go ahead, be your best
you know how, you've passed the test -
reach high, challenge yourself
blow off the dust, come off that shelf!
LLL

Did I really just type: I get gas? My, oh my!

Chapter 27 - Deepest fear

I have worked my way through this book, not preconceiving what I wanted to write, merely going through my 10 years of notes and letting them talk to me, then, touching the keys of the computer and saying "Come on fingers... express. Tell what you want to say." This writing wants to address my deepest fear.

It isn't fun talking about symptoms. Burdens. Medicines. MRIs, etc., but releasing this information HAS TO BE therapeutic. Even if it is draining while doing it. I feel many emotions writing. Vulnerable, being a biggy. But moreover, inspired to push through my fear and keep sharing.

While writing this, a surprise joy was having my daughter here and having a sleepover. Which was fantastic since she had moved out 6 months after graduating high school.

Having her here and then not - every other weekend for 3 years, (following the divorce) was always hard on my brain, especially Saturday mornings. Never sure if she was in my house or at her dad's. I always had to awaken and think... am I alone? Of course I have farm. With critters, you are never alone. But things like, one day your dad is at your door, next day, he has died and now your mom is in your house full-time. Confusing to a normal mind, if there is such a thing. Injured ... OY, YOY! Time gets over-lapped and mixed up.

I 'spose, as I get closer to finishing this book, I am feeling areas of my brain asking me to let go now. Let go of this past and get on with my life. This, I appreciate very much. It has been a heavy load to carry. Remembering brain injuries! Intentionally. Ik!

There has been this deep knowing that I would share something of value, if I did hold on.   So that part is good. The part that shook me so deeply, was what made me get up and write this at 2:30 in the A.M. It is amazing where fog can appear as we bust through to another level of being here.

The evening of our sleepover, I said good night to my daughter and went to bed. What a sweet night. I was a bit restless going to sleep. Not uncommon for me. But finally fell asleep.

I began having a dream.

The dream was very clear. I was with a new love. We were at a friend's house. We were alone waiting for her and her family to come home, returning with their son, whom I had not seen in many years, returning from Iraq. Suddenly we heard the door opening. "Surprise!" In walks my friend, her hubby, kids, family, their son, and so many.

I am hugging them all and I get to my friend's son, big hug, then I turn to introduce my new love to them - but I can't. I am blank. I am looking at him. His face gets concerned. My mind is blank. I keep looking at him. I feel full of anxiety. I search. I hope he will step up and introduce himself. I break out in a sweat and feel the room all go quiet as I try to remember his name. My LOVE'S name.   Oh my gosh. Remember, this *is* a dream!

The dream continues... the big, horrific blank space is there. I know him but what is his name? Help me! Suddenly, I look at him and say, "I am so, SO sorry. I am completely blank, forgive me."   Then I turn to all the quiet, worried faces, feeling for me and him - and I say, "This is my deepest fear. My worst nightmare.   Please excuse me, I am going to go to the back room and cry. I am so sorry."

The dream continues... my mystery love follows me in. I am on the bed crying so hard. He lays beside me. I am so afraid he is angry at me. I keep crying and saying, "I am sorry. I warned you about who you were falling in love with. I warned you." I look at his face and STILL cannot remember his name! I want to die.

Something in this horrific moment shifts. No, I did not remember his name. No, he doesn't hold me close and say, "It's okay baby, it is okay. I understand. Don't cry." Instead, on my own accord, I realize I am dreaming and with everything I have, I bust through the fog of the damn dream and wake up.

I laid there unable to move at first, realizing I probably had been holding my breath. I felt completely deflated and slowly awoke in the dark room feeling so sad. Then as I realized where I was, I opened my eyes and said, "NO!" I got up feeling horrible. Got some water. Remembering my daughter stayed and still down the hall. My gratefulness returned. I was still here. I remembered!

So now you know my deepest fear. Literally, what could be a screen play called: BEFORE SHE WENT AWAY, of a woman - after so many hits, wanting to glean TODAY! Love TODAY! LIVE today! Disappears tomorrow.

If you look up multiple concussions on Google, as I have mentioned before, doctors state that Dementia is way more likely to happen. When I read that, and when I watched the movie, Concussion, I cried quite a few times. But then, I snapped back into my body and said, "THANK YOU! This is what I needed to remind me to DO what I need and want to do while I am here!"

As I have said, this foggy journey - is hard stuff to share, but
***hoping* to bring *hope*!**

193

When dating a nice man earlier in 2016, for a brief time, trying to see if I could be okay with a relationship - I will never forget him saying, "My worse fear Laurie, as we get closer, is that some day you would wake up and not know who I am." That concern killed me. My stomach slammed hard. Because his fear was a valid one. My reply, "Well, is it worth it?" His fear spoke loudly to me. It did not take long before I ended that relationship.

That piece in my head, of not wanting to ever hurt anyone by loving me, opened up and said "NO." Don't let a love relationship in. No partner. Family and friends are okay, but not a one on one. Because, if this should happen, I would hurt the one I love.

I have read and seen the stories. The poor partner slowly becoming invisible right there in the presence of the one they love. And they cannot bring them back. All their years together, their memories, blank. Nothing. As I finish this book, it happened to my mom and dad. Dad, slowly faded away not knowing mom. It was horrible. For both of them.

When I watched the movie, The Notebook, I balled buckets. It was so powerful. Of course, thinking about my foggy brain on and off, over and over for 10 years - I think I locked something in that said, "You must go this alone." But then, as I shared in another chapter, a loving heart, who held on to the possibility of loving me, contacted me. Our window proved this heart can still love big time. And while it morphed into friends only, I am eternally grateful.

Like an angel that reached right through the thickest fog – during the time that my parents were both in my house, a man saying, " We have not met yet, but I AM STILL HERE, Laurie. I want to love you. I want to know you. I want to know what you have experienced so I can understand and support you. No matter how it turns out for us."

I think, in what we learned spending, 18 months

together, was major growing. And it was safe. We cared for and respected each other. It is really because of Michael's loving heart, I am writing this book. I wanted someone to know my journey. Thank You, Michael. Especially for all the love you poured out to my dad right til his last breath, holding me up as I fell.

I shared this *deepest fear* about love and forgetting - with a long-time spiritual friend. His exact comment back to me was, "I think something for you to consider is that some people would rather love fully for a short period than not to love at all, meaning that if someone loves you and your brain goes splat, then as long as they go in knowing the possibilities, let them - because you may give their spirit exactly what they took body to experience."

This made me cry. In an instant, my brotherly friend, Brit, Yogi Kai, brought me back to my core belief that we are spirits playing human, and our interaction with each other, has purpose. So get off my *insecure-for-hitting-my-brain* horse, and live, laugh, love and keep learning!

Just as my author friend had said how much she loves to *edit and edit,* and I said I *love to live it and write it,* we both are experiencing life, beautifully. Helping each other along the way. When we allow others in and give thanks for the blessing, even if the blessing is uncomfortable. Fog lifts.

THIS, right here, right now, as I write it and you read it - this is the stuff. This is the willpower to LIFT FOG. To have faith. Trust. HOPE. To know that you might be taken pretty deeply into fog. To see if you can remember.

You see, just because the fog lifts doesn't mean you will not get more fog! That is how we grow. But the secret, I think, is to remember the past foggy experiences, and declare: "I WILL BE OKAY! THIS IS OKAY! LIFT FOG... LIFT!"

Become AWARE. Present. Slowing down. Soften your

grip on the steering wheel of life. Dim your lights in thick fog, if need be. Yield to the right, on life's busy road, release fear, have faith and LIVE! Whoa. That was deep. Lol!

I think, with my deepest fear of losing my memory, it is the one reason I have been so proactive in researching about keeping the brain and body as healthy as I can. It is what keeps me taking Omega fish oils, Ginko Biloba, Folic Acid, Amino acids, Taurine, and everything else I can research to keep my brain from turning to Swiss Cheese and shrinking, as proven by science. And hey, if I said that already in this book, well, I repeated it on purpose or forgot. Either way, it is important information!

We take this beautiful melon on our shoulders for granted. We think we will get tomorrow to say: I love you, I am sorry, or how much someone means to us. Somehow, we believe that tomorrow will come and give us another chance. But the reality is, it might not. This might be it. Another hit. Brain checks out. But - we are here right now. Blaming another for THIS life, is a fog of its own. Lifting and letting go of blame, wow! HUGE!

This little piece ahead is a tough one to write but one more level to When The Fog Lifts. I have to end this with my optimistic, spirit-getting-a-human-experience *belief*, and that is this: *If I should mentally checkout before my body does, and I forget who my loved-ones are, I pray that I leave enough love and light for those to remember me by, and that this is not an accident, rather it is my soul experience to go through. Do not grieve for me. Embrace NOW. Treasure your beautiful mind. Use it, to bring love and hope to others. Be the change. We are connected. **Life is a gift**. OPEN IT!!*

Those last words just brought me the greatest comfort. THANK YOU dear WORDS. Thank you brain and fingers for working. THANK YOU God for letting me do this writing. Reckon ya don't want me home, yet!

NEEDY SHMEEDY

Dang I hate, when I catch myself
falling in to that trap -
of needing your love or approval
what a bucket of crap.

How do we get there, is it DNA -
from birth to needing others?
Is this really such a bad thing?
Maybe not - as sisters and brothers.

Maybe though - we just decide
too much pain - comes from this -
and so we isolate our heart
but inside, there's something we miss.

Well, okay, I can buy that,
and once again I will try -
to dare reach out - with heart on sleeve
man, I hope I don't cry.

But if I do it is because
I'm prying open my heart -
So here I am, this is me
creating a brand new start.

Needy Shmeedy, maybe not greedy
maybe it IS in our DNA.
To reach out and connect - with each other
and lift each other up - along the way.

Chapter 28 - Meant To Be

Anyone who has taken a few minutes to look around at the hardships, terrorists, hunger, poverty and so on in our world may have a pretty hard time looking at their individual experience in life and say: THIS MUST HAVE BEEN MEANT TO BE.

So when ya wake up to your life, and in my case, a farmer - critters depend you. You are divorced. Your daughter has graduated and moved out. You had to put your dad in a nursing home and felt blamed when he died, 23 days later. Your mom almost died 19 days after him with deadly Sepsis in her blood, then suddenly was in your care full-time. Spinning with exhaustion, grief, details, 2 homes, farm... to name a few. Oh, and my head that I smacked the day before dad died!

Life is not simple. Often, it is a lot of work. Aside from the obvious list, then there is plaino jaino farm life of hauling firewood. Getting firewood. Stacking hay. Dirt. Plants. Harvest. Farming. Burying dead critters. Elements of winter. On and on... There are days, I NEED a caregiver.

During days that I have awakened and could not remember the day before, or week before, like thinking I still had to get an MRI that had been a month before etc... it is freaky to ask, is ALL of THIS really *meant to be?*

While this book jumps around, remember, it is written by "moi" aka brain - scrambled-several-times, HEALING: Laurie. I can look back at this journey starting in 2008, bonk #1 and fortunate with notes, emails, and ways to remember, even through writing it in songs, I can share this stuff.

I think what I want to say here mostly, about "meant to be" is that we have choices: 1. It is all random. 2. It is God-divine orchestrated. 3. Predestined before we got here by choice. Or 4. Life is a dance that we do with the universe/God. Co-creating by waking up. Not just living like a puppet on a string. A robot. Instead, courageously facing fog to learn and grow. The last one, is different than *all* God-divinely orchestrated. Because to some, that would mean, you deserved it. Especially if you believe in a punishing God. Then your accident, loss, grief, anger, pain – might be blamed on God. Or the famously used: Matthew 19:26, Hallmark, check book and image sayings on GOOGLE: With God, *all things are possible.* Fog, gives us a chance to ask if it is meant to be.

This is such a touchy subject. I have no agenda here, to stuff a belief in your face. I am simply a survivor trying to take what I have experienced and thrive. Go higher. Go deeper. Go purposeful. Go wider. To step back and see what this brain injury and life is really showing me. In simply asking that question "is this meant to be?" Could I have signed up for this? That question has saved me from victim-hood many, many times. Student is much easier to understand.

I would like to think 5 years from now, I will be a very successful farmer growing for the hungry. Feeding the masses. Including many on this journey, not alone. Also that this book, and several others to follow, will be out there in the world inspiring whoever needs my words for encouragement.

My music will not have been left to gather dust on my shelves either. I will have reached higher, busted through FEAR. Busted through FOG. Busted through my FEAR OF GOOD. I will have risen with confidence and inspiration to sing. To speak. To write. To not question my abilities anymore. Heck, I might be an over-night sensation when I hit 60. A clear-headed, bright light! I'm workin' on it! Yahoosky!

I believe that the hits to my brain actually shined the

biggest light of all: *that we are what we think*. The melon on our shoulders gets filled with the stuff in Twinkies. JUNK. Stuff that can last forever and ever. IF, that is, we don't decide to get rid of the dark, negative power - that holds us down with FEAR.

One of my uncles ended up paralyzed for a year with a rare disease called Gulillain-Barre. Where the immune system attacks itself and your nerves, eventually paralyzing the whole body. This man, truly an extraordinary example of not giving up, was able, after a year on his back not moving, to come home from the hospital and from an electric wheel chair, gained back some feeling in his hands, able to talk and went on to build unbelievable works with wood. Bird houses, bed frames, life-like wood log trucks, on and on. And when you saw him, he would smile his glorious smile and hug you. An honor to hug him.   FOG and pain? You bet! Depth. OMGosh! Family support, amazing. His wife, my aunt DeEtta, an absolute unbelievable woman.

I say this story because my uncle was trapped in his body, flat on his back, unable to speak for himself, or do anything. He had to rely on everyone. So he was trapped with his thoughts. He is, by far, the biggest example of a spirit not convinced to just end and die with self-pity. Instead, believe, get stronger, and make time count. Build beautiful works of art. Love your family no matter how tired you are of the fight. What a lucky family, to know and love him.

My heroes: My dad and uncle Dean.

There is a metamorphosis moment sometimes with fog lifting. Rays of light streaming through. As if you can almost feel a choir of angels wanting to sing from the other side. At least, that has been this artist's view. But then, I really dig rainbows too. So I imagine the leprechauns are dancin' a jig when I get it! In my fog(s), when the sun has busted through the rain, bringin' a rainbow over my farm, I knew I would get better. HOPE remained.

If you are willing to go the distance, like in the movie, Field of Dreams, and believe, even just *attempt* to believe that your injuries, or your loved-ones injuries/fog, are not an accident. EVERYTHING being experienced is an opportunity to grow and learn. First off, it can teach empathy. In a split second, your injury lets you into the world of pain, loss, fog. In that second you can identify with many on this planet. Compassion can then grow from empathy. Empathy can help us know unconditional LOVE. THE KEY to an open heart.

I have to admit, in the thickest fog, I did not always have this clarity. How could I? I could not even tie my shoes without falling over. I stuttered when I spoke. I saw triple and could not walk as mini seizures would zap away my brain. My marriage collapsed because I could not handle living with someone who had to be right. Or - that is how I perceived him at the time. Going through a divorce, letting go of great health insurance, security, even a man in the house. My rock, who knew my stuff. It was scary as hell. Meant To Be? Yah, it was hard to say that at the time. But now, I have NO DOUBT. Without it, I could not have typed those last words!

Even being a single woman and the BS that can go with all of that, if you tend to be friendly. Men might be attracted and then what? Or you don't look injured, because you put on some make-up, smiled, and took migraine or seizure medicine, suffering daily. Masks to survive.

When I would get stuck in this fog - somehow my deeper self, would whisper to me. I would receive a song idea that in no way, shape or form, would my sound mind be able to create. But my foggy, altered-mind could! The repeating message I got over and over, was: LIFE IS A GIFT! Don't take it for granted. Fill your mind with GOOD. Release: FEAR OF GOOD/GOD aka F.O.G. All of these words that I type for you here on this page, to me, are gifts. Gifts BECAUSE of my injuries. Because of FOG lifting. Because, I believe I showed up here to learn. To repeat and learn and repeat and learn until I finally say, OKAY... I GOT IT! Now, USE it!

Even when the news, politics and opinions try to get through to my fear place, I now am looking at it more as a movie. A school. A college class. Asking myself, "Which way are you going to go on this, this time?" Full of anger. Hate. Jealousy. Forgiveness. Love. Joy. Fear? Am I going to cry victim? Can I look at every single thing and people involved with my journey as teachers? Maybe teach something back? WOW! Talk about a FOG BUSTIN' question!

If we were to close our eyes, and for a moment, be shown a pre-life. (Imaginations might be required here, but play along.) Perhaps we see ourselves as spirit energy, speaking with the Creator. A beam of light coming from a huge energy love light. (Or any form of the Creator that you might imagine.) Perhaps you have had one or many lives. Perhaps this is your one shot. There you stand.

Suddenly, the Creator asks you about your upcoming life. You are asked if want the whole enchilada or just a little sliver of being human? Do you want to be set up so you have to forgive? Set justice right? Speak up for the little guy? Experience rage? Kill? Be killed? Heal? Judge? Grieve? Love? Love unconditionally? Pain? Joy? Bliss? Connectedness? Creativity? Passion? Fear? Faith? Truth? It is your choice. But you will eventually need them all, to evolve ... Hmmm. *Tall order, Big Creator...* you think to yourself. A lotta work ahead if you choose the whole enchilada. Maybe just a lil' taco?

The brilliant spirit that you are, you fire back at the Creator: "So, will I like, get an A+ if I sign up for all that stuff and git'r done? How will I know, while I am being human? And then what? Do I get to return and stay on this side? Will I get bored? Be an angel? Learn to knit?" (Just seein' if you are payin' attention there) big Creator, God. The reply comes back: *"If you want to remember - while you are human, say it now and you will be given **wake-up calls** Simply tell the front desk!"*

Poof! You are zapped back into your human suit. Here and now, and we are yappin' about brain injury and lifting fog. You begin looking back at the trail of your life. Your progress. Your challenges. Where you are today. What you have learned about you, so far. Tiny waves of connection and understanding on a deeper level begin to pop through, until BOOM! There you are. You wake up. Right there, smack in the middle of being human. And rather than longing to return to home and the Creator - because life is too hard, you use these experiences... to find out, the biggest lesson of all: it is never us and them - it has, and always will be ONE. One big **US**. Suddenly you see the memo: *For your wake-up call: dial* **ONE**.

With that idea, coming back into your NOW of an accident. A loss. Many losses. Letting go. Looking at what you were doing and thinking before now. What are you going to LEARN from this? What are you going to DO with this?

If I brought this through well enough, then maybe "Meant To BE" makes a little more sense. If you read or look at anyone who has taken their big life changing injury, loss, event, and turned it into the highest good to serve humanity, by expressing LOVE, then, yah, it makes a little more sense.

I know this can be all be pretty hard to swallow. Especially if you do not operate from that part of your brain. Or simply, it makes no sense. I still chew on it all, in wonder and wonderment! Especially with devastation and suffering. But it feels possible to be true and gives ME hope. Because of that hope, you are reading this book.

Ooh la wee, tis meant to be -
that we are here, Sweet destiny.

Open the mind. Kindness is key -
to guiding the heart, Ooh la wee.

Ooh la wee, tis vital we see -
letting go of the past, we become free

To forgive the hurt that once owned me -
THIS is my new life, Ooh la wee!

LLL

Okay, so that was my little bit of trying to
sound like a wise, french poet. Or maybe...
just a lil tater. french fry!

Chapter 29 - Slow Computer

Tis 3:45 AM. My eyes are so tired that typing this hurts. Yet, lying in bed all night hurts too. So I got up. My dog, yawning loudly, is at my feet wondering why the heck we have gotten up so many times? Why I have tossed and turned so much?

I turn on the computer and it takes forever to come on. The circle spins and spins trying to open a screen. I watch this and reflect on two things: One, the previous day. Watching the rapid decline of my 83-year-old dad as Dementia suddenly made life a nightmare for my frail mama. Dad peeing the bed. Getting up to wander. Arguing with her and saying, " I cannot remember where I am." Sleeping, all day. Struggling to remember things. You find yourself asking God, "How long is the plan for suffering?"

Computer still trying to open.

More reflecting. Mom - angry at dad.   Seeing him in his jammies, he had on all day, going back to bed after being up only an hour or so. Dad angry that something is uncomfortable in his legs. You look and find his fleece jammies wadded up to his knees, under his jeans (for the few hours he was dressed) and a Depends brief on sideways.

I watched the circle on the computer going around and around. My computer, probably needing de-fragging, struggling to open up and operate. This, was my dad. Sometimes, me. Brain not working. Round and around.
Part two, I remember the horrible days following some of my

hits. Swollen eye lids. Stuttering. Tipping over. Unable to think. Brutal to track others' words. Not able to finish reading a sentence. Getting nauseous if I tried to write in cursive. Walking like a duck with knees buckling. Canceling appointments, outings and afraid to commit to most everything. Oh, and the headaches. The swelled fluid in the brain. Oh that pressure! The sense that my head was actually lifting off the pillows, while propped up, trying to sleep with the pounding headache. Waiting for morning to come.

Finally... the computer opens and I stare at an open blank, white page, right here, right before I typed this, wondering if I can share anything important with you. Stare. Stare. Fingers empty. Blank white page. I remember again the look in my dad's eyes that had been coming, since his stroke from 3 years prior. The laughter. The joy. The struggles. The fading. The blank stare. Struggling to open.

The little old man, who, one day, could be out running a chainsaw or tractor, while mom held her breath hoping he was safe. The next day, barely able to walk. Their painful disconnect marriage of 63 years.

My fingers start to type: 3:45 A.M. and here we go.

I think of me trying to decide if I can ever love again, have a job to survive, write this book, sing my songs, run a farm, or if, because of so many hits, will I slowly be that circle that cannot open up, like my computer? Slowing down to eventually a blank screen, and my loved ones will grow aggravated waiting for me to search for words, remember, try to answer. Blank white page. Can't open. FOG.

You see, in reality, I did not write this book for you. I did. But I didn't. While I hope and pray beyond prayers that one or two sentences will help you, bring you hope or comfort, in reality, I wrote this book for me. A mirror. Trying to understand. Trying to remember with the utmost gratitude of what I have come through. Asking, "Why?" But never asking, "Why me?" That part does not enter my brain, except to type it. I don't see myself as a victim. But as a student of life. Oh sure, when the head is so heavy you can't lift it, you feel a bit like you are being punished and someone will find you dead with a swelled head and grimace of pain on the face. BUT... oooh doggies when that fog lifts... gratitude comes pouring in again. If I could capture and bottle that pure joy - I would be a bazillionaire!

It is a bit odd, I must admit, how I have continued to take the course or class on "HOW TO BUMP THY HEAD MANY TIMES, AND LIVE TO TELL ABOUT IT!" Blank white screen at now, 3:55 A.M., filling up. Fingers working. YAY!

I think: YES, Laurie... I am using all the scrambled words up in my head, determined to take a nightmare and blessing and blend them together. This book. A smoothie! How cool is that! Keep going! (Little self talk there at 3:56!)

To give new meaning to a brain injury and spirituality, some how. A truth. Not just the images of many white lines of scarring on my MRIs, proof that I really did hit my head so many times. But, wanting some form of understanding.

At the end of typing this... daggum it... I will hit the little SAVE button at the top left of my screen. Otherwise, kind of like not paying attention to a big life lesson, it will be a holy shitola moment and all this typing will be lost. Forgotten. Gone.

Yipe, hitting SAVE, right now!

In reality, you reading or listening to this, if you are healing from one or more hits, stroke, or any huge debilitating challenge and fog - maybe surviving a day, an hour... we really end up with one constant... NOW. Then, that hour or day is in the past.

Surgery is a perfect example of this. You come out bandaged, swelled, medicated, pain... and you watch your body heal. The first few nights might be horrendous. But then it begins. Slowly, miraculously. We are unbelievable!

Even if I do not hit save and forget what I have shared, I believe that my soul is taking notes on a deeper level. It is trying desperately to remind me, to wake me up and bring me back to my biggest lesson of all: LOVE. Digging and asking myself if I am full of self-hate, disappointment, grudges? Feeling like I should suffer? Not worthy? Or, learning to LOVE.

Boy, when you start asking those DEEP and BIG questions, beyond headaches, tipping over, fog, fog, fog... it gets VERY interesting. It takes courage to ask. Depending, of course, on the severity of injury, some of this deep stuff cannot be asked or answered. The brain might be shutting down for reasons we cannot see. Perhaps it has been over used. Abused. Even *dangerously programmed* thinking.

Each time I reflect on this, and the many hits, I go back to one core question: "What was I doing, what was I thinking, when I hit? Was I days ahead of that moment? Or thinking about the past? Was I angry? Happy? Here is the biggy: Was I present? Life happens. We sure don't need a guilt trip to our soul that says, "Hey you, tis all yer fault because you were not present." Nope! That is not my message. It is just a lil' look back of how we might protect ourselves from now on.

Trick is, we have this amazing, unbelievable computer melon on our shoulders - that runs the whole show. Forward. Backward. Currant/present time. Once *hit happens*, ya can't go back. If we do, we will live with regret of the past. Ya cannot heal and let go, while living in the past. The fog, seems to me, like it arrives to help us get present. Giving us that experience. To use it and find a way to live a higher level of being.

So as not to add yet another pressure onto myself of, "Oh crap, now I am not being present enough" my only goal is to just try to be more aware.

In Yoga, besides stretching and strengthening, opening the heart/chest area as well as the pelvis area are a big focus. You are asked to become aware of what your body is doing. Feeling. What is your breath doing. Honoring yourself. Honoring each other. Bringing you into the present moment.

Meditation and prayer groups do the same thing. Church. Trying to glean from the moment with gratitude and mindfulness.

One thing I have learned, is that when I type, I have to be present with each word or I'll have to re-type it all again. Present, in that, I place my fingers on the keys, and let energy come through with highest good intentions. They are working with my brain. But there is something magical going on as well. It is a double meaning because I also try to keep my ego out of the way, that doesn't think it is good enough or second guesses my thoughts.

When I sing a new song, same thing. Old songs, like Stand By Me, that I have sung and performed hundreds of times, I can be thinking of my grocery list, and sing that sucker and no one would know. That is memorized in my cells, I guess. New thinking, new projects, new anything – can help bring the brain into present. It can be exhausting, but healing if we don't push too hard and create a whole new fog of OVER-trying. Or even bigger: OVER-thinking! Or OVER-OVER - scheduling! OH MY Gosh. I know this one very well!

My new NOW, is to try to check in with, well, NOW! Sounds like a new-age, far out and groovy riddle, doesn't it? But, when I walk into the low entrance of the chicken barn, or open a car door in the wind, or bend over near a shelf or table, by golly, I feel myself AWARE.   So, me thinks me hits are teaching me! I will fall short plenty, no doubt in other areas. But awareness is being present. I say use it!

Even with days of clarity – I go to bed every night and start over with some form of fog most every morning. My new focus is to awaken clear! As with the unknowing of the next day, each time I have written on this book, I have wondered if this will be my last entry. Of course, now you are holding this book. Reading it. So... obviously... I KEPT GOING. Woohoo!

Trust me, this is a weird way to live. Never with a complete view. A finished, accomplished project that is finally done, available to share. Instead, my projects feel like potential ... but in reality folks, that is life. We are the project. The *unedited* version. The beautiful imperfect perfection! We don't know how a new job, a child, a death – will be. We just try to show up as much as possible and experience.

As a farmer, I know that at the end of every growing season, we harvest, till under and let soil rest. Then, come spring, we start again. Every growing season and year are different, taking notes on the year before. Some are wet and seeds rot. Some are crazy hot and plants dry up. Some, bugs eat your crop, some are fabulous and bountiful. You try!

We keep learning and growing no matter what condition. Who is to say what really happens to the brain of Alzheimers. At least the soul. Does the brain shut off and head home with its soul, leaving only the shell of the body just waiting to shut down? Or deep on a cellular level, is the soul inside there still learning, or, perhaps teaching us - watching on. Trying to understand about our human fragile selves. The signing up ahead of time, to learn and serve? Perhaps?

*Deep in there, the knowing that we are spiritual beings -
going through this human stuff to grow.
Our true, authentic selves.*

What blows me away about this whole brain fading and/or injury stuff is: The scholar who suddenly cannot speak? The great athlete who commits suicide because of "the voices", the little old man who just one day does not know his wife of 60-some years,   checking out mentally, leaving those around them questioning: why and where did they go?   Like shadows on the wall.

How about those who hit, and a new being emerges? The black and white logical brain, suddenly full of color and art. The cold and distant brain, suddenly loving and embracing. The angry, suddenly grateful.

I think about the power of love and a smile. About grace. How I have tried to be kind. Gentle. In a family not always the same. I think about forgiveness. It has taken time and distance, but eventually returning to kindness. All the while, no one really knowing what has been happening between my ears, behind the smile. Until, this book.

Do you think we have the power to keep our brains alive, healed?   Do you ever wonder how much is about giving up to life? Throwing in the towel? Not just one or many injuries to the head, but to the spirit. The willpower to - keep on keeping on? Life can beat us up. We can give up.   I wonder that often. When I hear those younger than me. saying they had a "senior moment" honestly, I want to stop them. To say: Don't believe that! Don't feed that expression!

When marriages become resentful, one spouse may shut down. A living suicide. A way to say "I CANNOT DEAL anymore. I cannot process anymore. My computer is slowing down, crashing. I cannot find my way out. I give up. But I am stuck." How do we get here?   School of life?   Random?   Or, some weird way of actually waking us up if we answer the call? Again, asking, "Meant To Be?"

All I can say is, to the brainy, sharp, organized, detailed, info-filled, daily-planner adept, goal-oriented brains ... while I admire you and yes, sometimes envy you – don't forget to develop your heart too. Because if you ever take a hit, and that beautiful brain does not let you do the things listed above, all you will have as you go through the journey is, the heart. The place, not of thought processing, but the place of feeling. Where hope resides.

Any person that is still on the planet living with severe TBI, Cancer, any life-threatening condition - has to find a way to survive. To want to stay alive. The slow computer brain will run the show but the heart, an open heart, will cut ourselves some slack with grace and love. The heart will try to show us another level of life. A deeper reason why we are here.

The journey is the journey,
one step at a time,
we can use this moment
to be present heart and mind.
Or we can get to far in front,
then fall way behind,
oh the journey is the journey
taking one step at a time.
LLL

From a song on my
ONE TO ONE cd.

Chapter 30 - Horsin' Around

This title, is the title of a CD that I wrote and produced after one of the concussions. As I wrote it, I sadly looked out in a field with 5 big horses and 4 miniatures, unable to ride.

It was during a window, between concussions that I wanted to give my daughter the memories I had as a child. I rode all the time. Barrel raced. Gamed. Trails. 4-H.

I was a crazy bareback rider. Stuff like: jumping on my horse without fear, flying out of our driveway, down the country road, across the highway, and straight to the river. Jumping into the water at a dead run. No fear.

Fast forward, as a mama, trying to buy safe and sound horses for me, my daughter and then, husband, 'was a nightmare. We bought, sold, gave away, even buried 3 old-timer horses during a long stretch. Trying to find a safe horse for a head-injured person is a big trick. Horse traders, (true blue horse traders) tend to say some untruths to make a sale. So you have to go try them out. Risking injury.

Now, I am pretty bent on finding spiritual meaning as often as I can in all of this stuff. Sorry, if my mantra of spirit getting a human experience gets old, but it has kept me from putting a bullet in my brain when my brain wanted to quit. Remember this book is offering not only my journey in first-hand, but hope that it can inspire you - to lift fog.

So you have these big decisions to make on finding a safe horse. Then, if you get one, and it isn't safe, you have to find a way to find it a new owner. It was hard. The one mare that I did fall in love with, got a tumor in her stomach and had to be put down. Try saying goodbye to a Tennessee Walker named Ester, who I loved, was horrible. She was promised to be smooth as silk with her gaits and not to jar my head. I cried so hard I thought I would pass out. Even the vet hugged me. A non-hugging vet. All I wanted was something good. Gentle and healing. But the bigger terror was about to happen.

I healed some, and hit again. During post-hit, we tried to find a sweet horse for my daughter. We found a Welsh pony named Apollo. He was a doll. A little timid like someone had beat him. But easy to catch and willing. We were happy and hopeful.

On a sunny afternoon, my daughter and her bestie friend decided to play showmanship out in the field. We had pounded steel fence posts in and made a huge rectangle as a make-shift arena with rope. It was great. My daughter was in a pretty pink western shirt, her helmet on and started going in circles around her friend. Just like the real stuff. I was fogged-over, pretty big time. Tipping a lot. Had to use the hoe or stick for balancing myself. I was out in the garden, watching from all the way across the field. Filled with so much pride and joy to at last see my daughter doing this. Her daddy was home and in his shop.

Round and round the two of them went. I could hear her friend calling out, "Walk. Trot. Canter." All was going good. And then, my daughter stopped the little horse near the fence-line by the road, took off her helmet for a couple minutes, when a truck with debris in the back - happened to zoom by, rattling.

All the sudden Apollo bolted. Took off. I looked up and he was heading at a dead run toward the fence. My worst nightmare. Apollo turned right. My daughter went straight. Straight toward a steel fence post. No helmet. I screamed for her daddy. (My stomach is tightening right now.)

In a physical fog, not sure if I was running forward or backward - I ran to the field, her daddy right behind. He passed me by and got to our daughter, finding her face-down, not moving.   Strange how things stay in your cells. I am quivering as I type this.   Her daddy slowly rolled her over. She had not hit the fence post that was maybe 2" away, but was apparently knocked out a few minutes.

First he checked to see if she had hit her head. My fears raced. All I could think about was the paralyzed actor Christopher Reed who fell from his horse.   With a very dirty face, little tears, the words OUCH came as her daddy touched her arms and she became fully aware.

Finally standing up, very dizzy, they took her to the walk-in clinic, suspecting a broken arm. Sure enough, it was a fracture. But would heal. We still did not know how hard she hit her head on the ground. She did not complain about her head, due to arm pain. One tough lil cookie, she came through with wearing a sling for 6 weeks. No serious concussion. Other than her math became a struggle for awhile.

That changed the direction for horses for several years. We sold Apollo. Later learned he *had* been abused, and bolting out of fear was part of it.   Time passed, no horses, just minnies, and eventually, the pasture filled back up again with new saddle horses. Supposedly safe. Once again, I hit my doggone noggin. Yah I know. Sounds crazy. That is why I am writing this book. LOL! Now, I had hooves and try to saddle. Try to ride. But mostly, feel incredibly guilty that we had paid for horses we could not ride. My ex-husband was a trooper during it all. He knew my childhood joys. He knew what I was trying to do for our family. For my healing. Writing this now, I shake my head at it all. But fog can make you do some pretty weird things.

It wasn't until I found a special listing for a free horse named REO, a unique breed. A Bashkir Curly, that had been used as a therapy horse. The woman could not keep him. We went to look. He looked horrible. Skinny. Coughing. Snot coming out his nose. But so kind. So, so kind. She saddled him up, and when I got on, I could feel how carefully he stepped. Like he knew.

The former owner met us there. She is the one who found him originally and trained him to work with the severely disabled. The currant owner got him when the non-profit therapy Org. closed. She was sad to see his condition. He was unhappy. We brought him home. And for a year, Reo was a blessing. While I could not ride him much, I could safely work around him all the time. He didn't always get along with the other horses though. So that became an unsafe window.

In a flash, if you aren't familiar with horses, you can get squished in stalls and trailers, stepped on, bucked off, fall off, the spook out from under you, spin and kick another horse, and if you are there, you too, and so on.

It all came down to another hit, when another gelding we had in the field, who tended to be very busy with his head, swinging it back and forth - collided with mine. Another black hole concussion followed. Sadly, the more you hit, the faster symptoms come, and sometimes, worse.

When the neurologist looked at my, I think, 3rd MRI, and begged me to get rid of dangerous things like 1000 pound horsey friends, my heart sank.

I gave Reo back to the original owner, who put him back into service helping troubled teens in Redmond, WA. He became their rock star. I gave away the other horses to great people, and kept our 4 little minnies. Since then, I have had a few trail rides on a friend's horse, found out I cannot trot, for it rattles my brain too much, but nice walks on the trails is wonderful! For now, I am content to have my little horses as friends.

I called this Horsin' Around because of its meaning. To

some, it is what we did and got in trouble for - when we were kids. "Quit that horsin' around!"   To others, maybe, woohoo, makin' out in the barn. Giddy-up! For me, it was the desire, through the fog, to reach forward to something to live for. In my altered state, much like a football or hockey player who is injured, your common sense goes away, and your "I CAN DO IT" operates the brain. Back in the game. A dangerous place.

Depending how severe the symptoms.   As soon as I could walk straight without tipping over, or stop walking heel/toe like a duck... with knees buckling on me, my: I CAN - would come back. This, is why I have so many crazy stories. Why I would remodel my house, pull out and relocate big trees, way too heavy for me to lift, climb on the barn roof to seal it. And so on. Not because I wanted attention. Good heavens no!   Not because I wanted to impress. Hell no! It was because, I am a farmer. On a farm. Accidents happen. Life goes on. People need you. Your daughter needs you. Your parents need you. Your husband needs you. And then, you are alone and no help. And so on.

I had two choices, lay down, rest, try to heal, day after day after day... or, do what I could do for my sanity. It got me in trouble. Over and over. But – again, I am here.

When we go through this stuff, losing our common sense, losing our ability to do what we did "just fine" yesterday – the highs and lows and foggy in between(s) can really make you not want to wake up.

It is the pulling forth "something" that says, "this accident, is not by accident." The "horsin' around" kept me wanting to be alive.   Stepping back, when the fog lifts, you might find yourself, as I did, with way too many horses, or commitments, or appointments or regrets and slowly you once again have a chance to look at yourself and ask, "How did I get here again?"

If you asked my neighbors about Laurie Lee Lewis - oh

boy. They would have fun telling their version of visuals they have seen of this mud puppy farmer out moving and growing crops, tilling, planting zillions of flowers, vegetables for the food banks and usually grinning! Filthy dirty. Or freezing my butt off wearing my fashion-diva NOT, clothing ensemble of layers.

I fair to say, the example of my parents, working hard into their 80's, have been my motivation to keep moving. My crippled mama with no left knee. Bone inside bone, s-curve spine, beyond serious Osteoarthritis... out pulling weeds.

Right up til a month before dad died at 84, dazed and confused, if he could manage a wheel barrow, he would still bring in firewood and pick up weeds to help do his part, care for his wife. Even if he didn't know who *that lady* was.

So if neighbors described me, hmmm, I would probably be considered the dirtiest, hard workin' woman farmer, at least on our road! My daughter jokes that when I die, she will just bury me out in the dirt. All you will see is the toes of my rubber boots, with a painted rock:

> *"Here lies my mama. The real dirty girl*
> *in the soil for her soul. She loved dirt!"*

Anyone going through the fog, needs something. If you are severely injured and have to lie still, or quiet, this is critical. Eventually that "something" calling forth, will need to be filled to keep the spirit alive. Be it listening to talk/book/music CDs, programs, be read to, prayed to, sung to, anything as a way to express. Or, if mobile, even attending Traumatic Brain Injury circles or conferences ... to remind you that you and/or your loved one are not alone. There were days, I would literally lay down in the dirt. Dig my hands into the new soil, deeply. Trying to ground and find myself.

I cannot say enough, about patience and time as medicine. Herbs, vitamins, nutrition, exercise, fresh air, and hydration. One note on water: If you can smell your water, aka chlorine, get a filter! If you research the damage of chlorine – you will see why! Also, be careful with the doctors and neurologists that you go to for HOPE, for they may not give that to you, partially because most of them have not had an injury.

I will also repeat: if you hit... **tell someone**. Watch for symptoms. It is hard to track this stuff when you are the brain going into the fog. But there is a critical, dangerous window, especially in the re-hits. Get to ER if you have symptoms. *Please.*

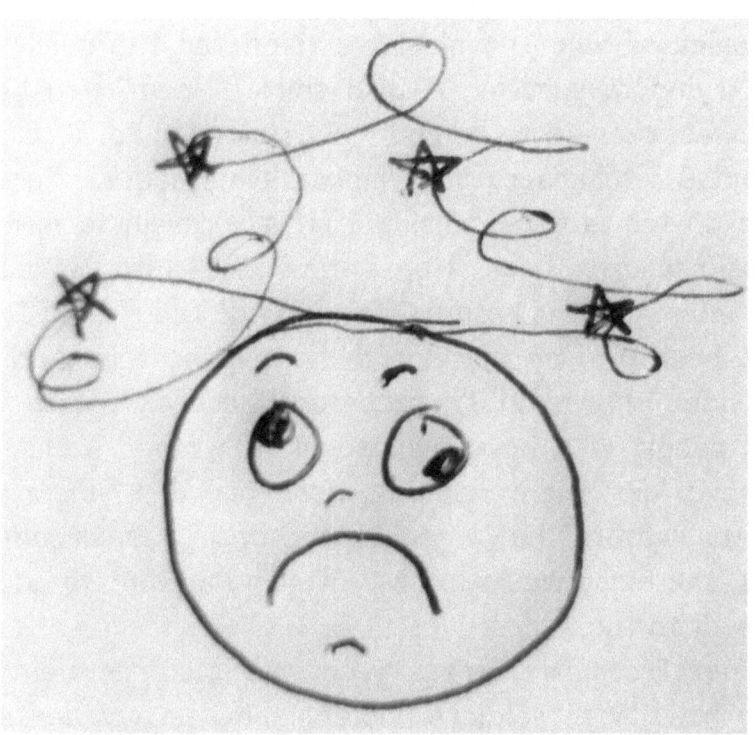

Chapter 31 - Ya booze Ya lose

As at least I *think* I mentioned before: the constant companion of "Did I say that or just think it really hard?" I have mentioned when brain injury has happened, often a doc will prescribe meds to help you sleep, stay calm, refocus, fight depression. All challenges! There is a lot of talk and discovery about marijuana for the pains and migraines and anxiety that can come with brain injury.

In attending 2 brain injury seminars, I heard quite a few stories of what people have tried for the quick fix or simply trying to survive. I also think I mentioned beer, in small doses, seemed to helped me. Calm my mind. It is full of hops and B vitamins so that makes some sense. Pure hops extract or tea is very calming. It is a cousin to marijuana. Makes sense. Into beer it goes, beer goes into us, buzz and mellow fellow are the result OR... sloshed! The FINE LINE!

I hesitated on writing about drinking and head injury but decided it was VERY necessary because I have known several people who have bumped and thumped - and drank. They have lost their families. Bank accounts. Licenses. It stands to reason, that when a poor brain has already been altered, the biggy would be, why would you want to add more disconnect to the wiring.

Post Traumatic Stress Syndrome is so prevalent in our country now. With soldiers, violent families, accidents... the list is long and we are the most medicated country in the world.

I called this, ya booze, ya lose - for a very important reason. I am a light weight anyway so booze is pretty low on my list. Yes, now and then a good beer. But when you are struggling to heal, this again, is your wake-up call opportunity to either medicate heavily and mask your journey, "wallering around in the doom and gloom" or medicate lightly as possible, to calm the neurological symptoms, as you get stronger. Focus on lifting fog - instead of creating more.

Again, if you are reading this as a loved-one, you are trying to understand how you can survive and how you can help your loved-one. Knowing they are already altered, you may have to intervene and help them try to see this journey... of what is happening to them and why. As the injured brain, most of the time, the fog is too thick to even be able to get that far on your own.

In fact, you might be the golden light or messenger that will help the injured one go much deeper than the brain. Into the heart and soul! This journey will be your journey too.

I just have to add, as I clip along here, and I try to keep up with my fingers - that if you are the caregiver or loved-one caring for someone altered, this is NOT easy. It is NOT fun. You could be feeling punished yourself, for having to stick it out. I just want to say, from one who has carried guilt for feeling like a burden - **THANK YOU** beyond words. You too are learning what happens when the brain doesn't function correctly. When all hell breaks loose for us, the injured one, YOU the rock that we turn to, are so appreciated. Even if we the injured forget or cannot tell you! **THANK YOU**! But please remember yourself. That whole self-care tag that is now being said on news and pamphlets IS true. Hard to do. But critical for YOUR sanity!

We are always just a blink from role reversals. Sometimes needing to help another, sometimes needing the help ourselves. Like alcoholics that stop drinking and find out who their real friends are, this stuff will bring out EVERYTHING.

Some people will avoid us. Others try to help by finishing your sentences. Others talking as if it could never happen to them, and then ... whammo. Game over on the count of brain pain.

The injured brain and the caregiver need to find ways to stay strong. So rather than lower your immune system with booze, consider drinking, for health sake, ... smoothies! Fill your body and brain with as many amino acids, vitamins and minerals from veges and fruits as you can. Even if you can buy a powder loaded with all of that... YOU are worth it.

Cutting back on sugar is helpful too. Helps the highs and lows calm down. WATER is mega important to keep the brain hydrated. Now remembering if you have *had* any water or not – that can be a big stinker challenge, at least for me. So I have found that a pitcher or quart jar that says DRINK THIS helps. Anything. Adding a little lemon is nice. I find I drink more of it. Or, hot water with lemon. Herb teas. FLUIDS! A thirsty brain is a foggy brain.

Ha! I have no idea what I will be sharing next... but anything that I can remember in this LONG journey back to wholeness will be written. I am willing. Hopefully, I will share something of this mongo soup of thoughts... that will help you on your journey too! MMMM soup. I must be getting hungry!

Chapter 32 - Must Be Present to Win

With all of the head thumps, I have never asked, "Why me?" I knew why. I was in a hurry! Head anywhere but present. A list in my head of: to-do-its. Not mindful of where my mind/head were! Nothing wrong with that, but I tell ya what, once Thumper thumps... and you are suddenly on the journey back to "quality of life"... it forces you and/or your loved ones to say "Watch your head."

You find out quickly if you will listen or ignore. Listen or ignore. Repeated there on purpose. Um, speaking from personal experience on this one! (She says with a smidgin' of guilt.)

But, what if... the track we are on, the zipping around, all the goals, the gotta be, gotta do, and such, suddenly got put on pause? Yup, pause. Someone reached through the ether or ozone layer (since it is getting so thin now) and hit your pause button. WHOA! Freaky, stinky, whoa!

In fact, maybe you could barely see, but life might suddenly look like a surreal cartoon show. EVERYONE going, going, going. Bitching what they had to do next, school, love, work, taxes, gas prices, weather, holidays, bills, money, bad drivers, crowds, politics, traffic, slow lines and so on. You just look on, but can not enter in. Hmmm. As a friend of mine use to say in his talks, "You stood back and watched the yes and no - chasing each other around! Never happy."

This is why it is so popular to get stoned. Drunk. High.

Wasted. Whatever you want to call it. It detaches you from the cartoon show. You don't fit in. You are too slow. Numb. It is almost funny. "Like... Dude, like, whatever... what's the hurry, man. Chill out!" What someone says, zings right past you. While I covered this on *Ya booze, Ya lose*, there is more.

When I attended the TBI conferences in Seattle, both times I heard the most incredible stories. Horrific too. Blessed. Angry. Some, incredibly grateful. We were a whole bunch a dents in one big motel. It was awesome and of course, sad. I am surprised they didn't hand us all big pom pom wigs to wear as a symbol of protecting and respecting our beautiful minds, as we cheer-leaded ourselves into the courage to heal.

What I saw was many smiles. Hugs. Walls and barriers gone. Grateful to connect and hear stories of encouragement. Things like: "Any chance this was meant to happen?" Oh man. If you ask that to some people that are in serious denial/victim, why-me mode... this will piss them off big time! But they are entitled to that anger. Cuz there's a whole lotta foggin' goin' on upstairs! They do not, nor should not be rushed to answer that question.

There is a lot of hell that goes with not being able to speak, stand up, compute. It is terrifying, frustrating, and the world keeps turning fast, whether you are altered or not. In fact, people in your life may stop coming to see you. May be impatient with you. May call you a fake. Lots of stuff, besides pure survival mode. Anger of limitation is very normal. Lecturing the injured one to "Come on, at least you are still alive, could be worse." While one is still in that angry zone - it probably will not help.

Me, being a spiritual chickie poo that thinks I am a spirit here on earth getting human experiences for soul growth, be it one lifetime or many... well, I went through all of the emotions. But, when the fog lifts, I remember my core belief, that this is *my* journey to *grow*. The minute you decide and choose direction, fog begins to lift.

The kicker of doubt says: Yah but, I did it over and over and not just bonkin' my brain. Marriages. Moves. Surgeries. Attracted abuse. Many jobs. Lots of let downs with music. No money. Over and over?   Really? Soul growth? What? Was I an absolute idiot that signed up on the other side, askin' "Hey awesome CREATOR OF ALL, could I please have a lifetime, that feels like about 50 in one?

While I wrote on this already, I think, didn't I? (I really want to keep reminding you of who wrote this book!) LOL! And because this angle to the fog lifting has helped me, I will repeat here. Food for thought.

Back to GOD: *So, at warped speed - you give me all the emotions I can handle. You place me perfectly in a family, where I am sure to have very low self-esteem, maybe give me a gift like music, in a reasonably attractive body and trusting heart and then - see. Just see if one of your kids can remember that I am a spirit that came here to get all these wonderful experiences. Then, hey God, while we're a chattin here... if I am a good spirit and remember and wake up - can I have a pony with a pink mane and tail that flies? A safe one? Ah, just playin', God, I have 3 miniature horses presently, and they are wonderful!*

So MUST BE PRESENT TO WIN... you cannot go back in time. But you CAN remember. You CAN honor, celebrate, learn-from or get stuck in those memories of the past. You CAN choose to forgive and let go of the past. You can always distract your current life with the visualizing and focusing only on the future. Or fog-out with booze, drugs, TV or ???

All the information on the LAW OF ATTRACTION talks about this stuff. "Telling the universe what you desire. Place your order. Live like it is done. Have faith. It will find you. Then think about it again and again and again.   Then, let go. WHEW. It is fun and gets you asking: WHAT DO I WANT?

But the bigger, deeper message is actually: get clear what you desire, and then, *let go of that control.*

If you do the *future living* or the *past*... then the life in the NOW passes you by. Your head is set on back or forth but not in the middle NOW. So when the drawing of the raffle ticket brings up your number that says YOU MUST BE PRESENT TO WIN - and you popped out of the room to go check your phone. You were bored. You were bitterly sick with disgust about a family or friend or elections or ? That winning ticket, that little girl saying "daddy/mommy, will you play with me? A phone call from a friend you cannot pick up, etc... THOSE GIFTS are the winning ticket.

I find that when I really try to live as present as possible, dang, little things like going to the post office or store on errands, little sparkles of *cool* tend to show up.

This stuff happens when I can bring my focus into NOW, this place. Not living in the past. Thinking too far in the future.

Hangin' in the now, man! High on life and getting another day.

Sadly, we have created a world of foggy attention disorder. Not all of us are on meds for this, but we can certainly understand when life gets multi-directional and hard to keep up. Especially after injury! Makes it very hard to be present.

What is that saying?

THE PRESENT -
ISN'T THAT WHY THEY CALL IT A GIFT?

Chapter 33 – A WHOLE NEW FOG

While this next chapter includes fog... as you will soon read, this type of fog for women is brutal! Amazing we don't have more serial killers that are women. I have always thought God had a nasty sense of humor giving us periods, PMS, Menopause, hormones, innards trouble, surgeries and the birth machines for life!

Following Hits 1, 2 and 3... in 2008 things were rough. Can't say a whole lotta genius or "present" was going on.

But by Spring of 2009, I was planting a garden again and kinda back to me. Mostly. This whole head thangy was new and maybe I was a little more careful. But not physically. I am a tree-movin, dirt shovelin' queen. I love using my body physically. My daughter would often say, "Eeeew, mom, your biceps are like camel humps! That aint right!" Hehe. What can I say.

But my oh my, the: *when-is-enough* "common sense" just wasn't there. My pain tolerance had gone way up. After-all, I endured some big uglies for months. Headaches for weeks that would literally feel like my head was going to explode. Mostly I had to sit up at night on a couch and find one 1/8 of an inch left or right to place my head for a bit less pain, to try to sleep. Even hydrochodone did not help. Nasty. I tried a couple migraine meds too, but they made me woozy.

Soon as those stinkers would leave, I was on fire to DO STUFF. Workin' on the farm, I never knew when to stop. I was just so happy to DO. It felt so good.

2009 was my celebration. I had not hit my head for almost a year! YAY ME! Reports about concussions said that there was often a big fog-lifter, about a year following. Oh, and my music was coming back as well. After the 3 hits, I could not sing my own songs for months. Hundreds I have written, just left my soul. It was very sad to be that disconnected from my passion. But I could slowly start singing old standards again, like Lion Sleeps Tonight. That was good. If I forgot the words, I wasn't performing, so that was okay. Horses didn't care! All was going very good. Family dynamics good. Even camping entered the picture. SO GOOD.

Well, come summer, my good fortune ended. All because of my stubborn self. While pullin' out a cedar tree which had a whopper root ball. (My on-going joke is that when trees see Laurie coming with a shovel, they grab their root balls and hold on tight!) Sorry, had to include that here. Cuz its true! Unless they are female.

Well, shovelin' and pullin', suddenly I had the sensation of a bowling ball in between my legs. Sorry fellas. This might get a little gross. But hey... life happens, even when you aren't havin' fun! The pressure was like something had been torn loose up inside me, and the discomfort was unbelievable. I was instantly nauseated. Getting to the house to lay down was a struggle. Soon as I laid down, the pressure would stop. "Cool" I thought. Let's get back to it.

Soon as I stood up, boom, that horrible pressure was back. Now this was about June. Garden all up. Lookin' great. So can you imagine, to finally be able to bend over without my head going nuts, totally blissing in dirt... suddenly I could not barely walk out to see my beautiful garden.

I made an appointment with a walk-in doc. A young man. I told him about the pressure. I said "nothin' has fallen out, but feels like all them female parts are hangin' by a string." He listened to me, then kinda uncomfortably asked, "Well, do you want me to look and do a pelvic exam?" At some point, after dealing with this for a week, I wanted to yell: "Hell yah!" But I was a lady and said, "Um, yes, that is why I am here, thank you." (Like I WANTED to be there. Grrrr...

The doc was nervous. Maybe cuz I was so beautiful. Bahahah ha! Not! A nurse came, we did our lil giddy-up stirrups and he said, "I think you have a prolapsed uterus, falling. But I am not positive." I took this inspection story and before I got in to a specialist, I think I saw 2 more doctors - it was nuts!

Finally after weeks of discomfort, the specialist, who was originally from Ukraine, came in looking like Star Trek's young Chekov. Seriously! As he came in the room, first thing out of his mouth glancing at me, was: "pretty" as he came around to make eye contact. He then asked me why I was there. I tell him "Prolapsed Uterus. They think." Explained the horrible discomfort, etc.

He listened and then came back in his strong Ukraine accent with, "Who tell you, you prolapse?" Again, I say, uh, 3 docs. 1 walk in, 2 family. He looks at me like I am making it up. "We take a look" he says.

Through my knees, I hear, "Okay, you prolapse. You have big problem! More than uterus." And then came the kicker: "So... I feeex. (fix) We give you hysterectomy. I take out uterus, left ovary, feex 2 tears." Then, he asked, "How many children you have birthed?" I answer, "one." He looks up through my knee caps window, and replies, " Must been terrible birth, yes?" I say, "VERY."

It took until September to get the surgery. Two months! My garden was huge. Bountiful. I had to lay down to pull weeds. A neighbor came and helped me. She felt so bad. I was so grateful. I knew once I had surgery, life as I knew it, would not be the same. Especially the first 6 months. So much for fun garden and healed-brain summer!

The "I FEEX" did 4 things. I had stitches everywhere on the inside and out. I don't need to tell ya, I was one hurtin' woman. They did not tell me, that I would basically be tipped upside down for over 3 hours. But boy, on top of the surgery, I remember horrible headaches following the hysterectomy. I now was hollow. No ovaries (had right one removed a few years before do to bursting cysts) and no Uterus.   Hollow mama!

As I healed, what I did not reckon with was the fact that there would be NO hormone production. All my energy from my being had suddenly gone to heal this horribly invasive surgery. I felt lost. Confused. Like a big, fat concussion with stitches!

Months past and moved into 2010. I celebrated one part of this whole thing... well, two. That dang bowling ball pressure was gone. The rest was hell, but eventually in months to follow, I sealed and healed!

But no hormone production was not cool. Suddenly, I went from zipping woman who moved trees and healed from 3 head hits in 2008, to menopause, hot flashes, mood swings, no sleep, chills, one very confused woman. I repeat... I felt lost.

But... and it was a BIG but... I did not HIT MY HEAD. In fact, I was starting to sing again. And strum my guitar more and more. Even some of my songs were coming back. Previously, I had sung a lot with my daughter and her daddy. We were called Calico Hearts and folks knew about this sweet little family that sang nice folk/country/inspiration music. But when I bonked, we disappeared. As I got stronger, that part returned and we once again enjoyed our music for a window.

Now it might seem odd to share this window about hysterectomy in a brain injury journey book. Especially if you happen to be of the feller type asking "and how does this fit in?" Well, fellas, you have no idea what happens when hormones that operate a woman through their life - to be WOMAN, suddenly are not there at all. You thought PMS was bad! You take ovaries out of a woman, she cannot produce the hormones that create health, good bones, mental balance and a list off the page.

Gals, oh my gosh, we know this is an entire, huge world. As we go through natural or forced menopause, the brain fog can be extremely thick. Sleep completely screwed up. Emotions off balance. Weight gain. Depression and the list goes on.

As I write this, I am reminded back of what Dr. J tried to tie in with my concussions, that it may have JUST been menopause. While his statement of menopause was true, his ass-ssement of me was way off! This was definitely trauma, body, mind and spirit.

Something worth mentioning, regarding hormones, if you research, you will find that concussions, dementia, stroke, can also have an extreme effect on hormone production. Men too! Testosterone can drop significantly. For women, especially if the area is near the Pituitary gland.   Or, from a hit, a woman might start producing estrogen and suddenly, emotional sides may come out - that were not there before.

It is fascinating how we are wired together. But add a hysterectomy, it gets so crazy. No ovaries. No hormones. Without supplementing somehow.

I really did think about whether this chapter was worth sharing. This book is called WHEN THE FOG LIFTS and for every woman reading this with or without brain injuries and have gone through PMS, pre-menopause, or flat out - the boom of Menopause. YOU KNOW the fog!   You know when something is operating your being that was not there before. Fortunately, there is help with menopause and hormones.

About 5 months after the hysterectomy, inflammation took over my joints. I was a mess, aside from sleep, mood, etc.

My doctor put me on Premarin to see if it could help. Omgosh! I got a whopper 5-day migraine. Then learning about how Premarin is extracted inhumanely from pregnant horses, I just could not do it ethically. I was getting depressed thinking I was stuck like this.

Researching, I discovered Bio-identical hormones, that, while my insurance would not pay for it because it was considered natural, I could get a prescription. My family doctor worked with me. Over the next few years, I took them.

This inflammation condition actually had awakened right after I had given birth in 1998. My hands would not work. Slowly as my hormones restored, I got better. Now, suddenly all my joints stiffened and were inflamed again, post-hysterectomy. I swear by the bio-identical hormones. They saved me.

Besides the hormones, I also detoxed, cut out all kinds of foods, white sugar/flour/rice... anything to try to combat this condition. I found corn, salt, MSG, pork, nightshade plants like potatoes, tomatoes and peppers and of all things, ice cream, to be major culprits. I am pretty careful now.

Once again, I share this stuff, because it was a fog that moved in so thick that I thought I would be a cripple for the rest of my life. I still carry this condition, and get reoccurring symptoms if I don't keep my immune system up.

With the history of injuries to my brain, plus radical Menopause, I look at all of this as the rites to passage into a wise woman. The jury is still out on how wise, but dang! If you can survive it, and all the physical changes that we gals go through - essentially ladies, we are QUEENS. God bless the menopause woman!

On that: just as FOG can be thick for the first month after giving birth, with hormones all whacked out a place, post-pardon blues, sleep deprivation, engorgement, etc. I say:

GOD BLESS THE WOMAN WHO BIRTHS THE CHILD.
Holy Shhhhhmolies ... If we can endure childbirth and menopause... we should be running the world! Sorry boys, but it is true! God made us strong!

I guess I am trying to lay out a visual here that says, you might be going from one condition to another, as I have. Each with its own fog.

Put all of that together and then add - the latest discovery: THYROID. If thyroid is all off balance, that too creates fog. I know some people are taking a tiny dose of iodine. Or adding Selenium and Folic acid to their daily vitamins, and seeing/feeling a significant change. FOG is FOG. Figuring it all out... is a pain in the butt. Hey, I did not say ass. Pretty good huh?

My dad, with his post-stroke/dementia window was trying these supplements. It was hard to know which was the actual hero of the day when dad had a clear window. And then, he was gone again. But the idea that hormones and thyroid are connected, it gives another door to open and research if you haven't done so already. Includes both women and men. You may have to be pretty insistent to your doctor though.

It is exhausting. I admit, I have been more than willing to open my cupboard, take down my DHEA which I now take instead of bio-identicals, my Ginko Biloba, my selenium, folic acid, and mega oils... I am happy to swallow most every day in HOPE that it will protect my brain. Rebuild the damage. Head off Osteoarthritis, that has devoured my mom. TIME, HOPE and certain supplemental help seems to be working.

As I stop here, pause, and ask, "ah Laurie, (self talk is okay if positive) what was your intention here on this chapter? Pause. Meno – pause ... Mental - pause.

Aha! A piece of my brain just kicked in to remind me as I work hard to type, re-type and share all this stuff. This is a bit like droppin' all your clothes, and headin' bare-ass naked down on the road, past all your neighbors, into the bank and grocery store and every other place I have been, including the stage... and saying, "Yup, this is me. This is what is under what you have seen."

Another part of my brain kicks in to reality, laughing at itself to say, "Laurie, I know you mean *HOW VULNERABLE* you feel to share all of this about yourself, but woman, think about it! You described your other image of you bare-ass naked on the road. Talking about your brain injury journey is nothin'! No worries, girl! Gidd'r done!

Menopause, mental pause
show me God - in life's clause
why on earth WE gals must birth
little humans, bring em to earth

Oh and Seriously Creator God
You wired man oh so odd ---
he can't wait - to get back in
to that sacred space - some call sin!

So hey there God, give us a break
lighten the load - in this big ache
boys would faint to deal with this stuff
Holy Moly, we gals are tough!

And so its time to campaign
put a woman in charge with heart and brain
She's earned her place - she knows her stuff
yup like I said, we gals are tough!

Chapter 34 - Profound Horse shit!

So how ya doing on this ride with me? Is your butt getting' saddle sores from all my yappin? Mine is! I hope I am bringing some humor and insights to you.

Well, this should be a "gooder" as dad would say. Let's see what the fingers type. Giddy-up:

As a farmer and cowgirl, ya watch where ya step! While horse turds stink up your shoes, they also fertilize your farm! Right at this moment... you are probably saying GROSS and/or shaking your head saying, "WHHHHHAAT?!?! Stay tuned. Ride along...

Farm life, "livin' the dream," isn't always pretty. I have put down and buried many animals. Held them as the vet injected euthanasia medicine. Down they went. Pain over. (Of course I balled buckets of tears every time.) The path up to the pinnacle "pain over moment" may have been days, weeks, months. Decisions on who should live and who should not or when, is nuts on the brain and worse on the heart! Stir that in with concussions, yah, SO not fun.

As ikky as it may sound to read that last paragraph, well, when it comes to your beloved father, mother, family, or friend - we humans do not have that option legally, unless we go to certain places in the country or world. There, you, yourself, and doctors orders, can pay and fulfill your choice to die. Here, we only have the choice of suicide. Or wait it out. Weird huh? And, most of the time, suicide is perceived as such a warped method of checking out - *most* of the time. Unless you are totally gone. Or watch someone starve to death because while their mind seems gone, their body won't die. Even worse if they ask you to help them, and you can't!

They do surgery, knock you out, remove body parts or add some, and then you wake up and take pain meds - til the pain gets better. But dying can be like some birth, extremely painful. Slow. Get stuck. Life support keeping someone going. And so on. However, it seems with dying, the soul kinda has its own agenda. Some hang on til everyone pops in to say goodbye. Some die quietly after everyone leaves.

Thanks to Hospice, and their access to drugs, many can have Morphine to exit the body with less pain. But certainly that is a minority in our world. When dad was in the nursing home, a nurse told me that people and animals will often naturally stop eating and drinking to shut the system down. And, though I do not know how they prove this, the nurse said that after the initial discomfort of this act, the body apparently begins to produce an anti-pain endorphin. Boy I hope that is true!

I guess unless you die and then can come back to tell us this, we really just speculate. I WANT to believe it. Especially for all who suffer.   Especially saying goodbye to my dad, my dog, my horse, cat, and blind chicken – all, in less than a year. One dramatic 2018 stretch! Yipe!

Our experience with Hospice wasn't quite to so pleasant. They took over dad's care one month before he died. The challenge was, that once dad went to a nursing home with Dementia, dad's "caged animal" aggressive state grew. His natural instinct was to fight the medicines being prescribed. For any of you reading this who have had to be the one to place your parent or grand-parent in a nursing home, there is nothing more brutal. Guilt is the worst fog.

While I do not hold Hospice accountable for dad's

death/exit, I do have concerns about the voice of family when Hospice takes over. There seems to be a big disconnect with doctor, nurse, facility, family. What I experienced was a battle. To my knowledge, in 23 days, dad was not seen by an actual doctor. Only medications were prescribed by Hospice to ever-changing nurses.

I learned that when Hospice takes over your loved-one's case, your family doctor disappears. Hospice will do this if they think the person will die within 6 months. Most of the time, the stories are amazing. They come in and you receive whatever is needed for "comfort care" for your loved one and your family too. They get paid through insurance and DSHS.

Sadly, dad was over-medicated with various sedations - until his death. I believe he had 5 meds in him. I fought. I pleaded. It was hopeless. At one point I had to tell the facility *HE WAS NO LONGER SWALLOWING* as he choked on medicated applesauce! When my brother found him on his knees frozen by his bed, it was too much. To me, it was a horrible death, but then, death comes in many packages.

The only grace that came from this nightmare was the day we had to move dad to a second facility because he hated the first one. When he realized he was not coming home, he got very upset. I wanted to put him in my car and go home. I hated it. My guts hurt so bad. I finally broke down. Then, in dad's agitated state, which soon would get worse, he saw me. He came back into his mind long enough to put his hands on my face in the hallway and say "Oh Sis, I am so sorry you are the one that has to do this. I am so, so sorry. It will be okay!" We held each other and both cried. Just typing this still makes my guts ache and tears. 16 days later, he was gone. Having a walking Dementia patient is not easy for a facility if they get agitated.

It seems the sum total of that last couple months with

dad's decline – gave me words to write and share here. Insights. I hated this experience. I wanted to run. Oh my gosh. Or hide. Or have a nervous break-down. I could not cry deep enough. I literally felt my guts in my belly button tighten and bend me over with pain. I was so surprised. I thought surely I would just spiritual-up on this whole page. Not! But I seem to be a conduit of experience = words = this book or song. Trying to express and help others. So here's what wants to be written without me deciding if it should or shouldn't be:

Since this book is about busting through fog and my journey through brain injurie(s) – thinking that I was near the completion of my story, well... suddenly I walked the walk with my dad's death. Dad not only had Dementia, he also a frontal lobe tumor, plus a stroke 4 years prior and concussions before that. Plus, severe toxic poisoning lung damage in 1982- and as a child, Rheumatic Fever twice, bedridden for a year. Quite a man. And, until I was around 19, his alcoholism dominated, til he quit cold-turkey. Quite a ride. For all of us!

Through all of it, dad showed/taught me something. Stay authentic. Work hard. Do your part. Enjoy little things. Don't take life for granted. At his earthly end, it came down to a smile. A word. A song. A touch. At the end, I found myself getting close to his face and saying: "Hi daaaaad and would sing softly" to bring him back to tracking me, when he was glazed over. It would work every time til the end. I cherish those memories.

At one point, dad took my hair that laid softly on his face, and held in over his eyes. I felt like I wanted to go with him. I did not want to stay behind. My brain. So much. Mom. Our family. It was me that had to do the hard thing. I had to put him in the facility. It was me he begged to take him out.

During the daily spiral of over-medicated, shutting down, fighting the meds, his spirit tried to hang on. I would gently touch his hand and face. I could feel his muscles appreciate that tenderness. I told him GOOD JOB over and over. That he did a GOOD JOB as dad. The work was done. Very well done.

While my folks hung out for 63 years of marriage, like many long-term relationships, affection was not always there. My mom traveled a hell of a road with dad. His caregiver, wife, friend, singing partner and sounding board for a lot of, as she called it "shit fit" swear words. Yup. Dad could string words together that could make you cringe or laugh - if you could disconnect from it. Usually brought on by his severely painful body trying to do his part, his fair share or inability to think or injury. So many injuries.   Low income stress. So much. Mom's medicated brain made her hyper, which was even worse for dad.

I walked eggshells often trying to create an aura of protection for my dad. That was exhausting. Amazing what love will do.

So you are probably asking why the heck did I call this chapter PROFOUND HORSE SHIT?   Sorry, if you are trying to walk a very religious/dogmatic/squeaky-clean perceived path and knee-jerk at my language, well, I am my father's daughter. And now that he is ethereal, on the other side of the thin veil of spirit and human, I really am not worried what others think. Whoa, did I just type that? I need to write this page down! Might need it again, like... tomorrow when I forget! Ha!

I found myself during the journey of helping dad (mom too) ... actually telling family "I do not care if you love me or even like me." Try saying that once. It is so wild. Freeing! **WOW! 56 stinkin' years to get that out of my mouth!**

Trying to please my family. Trying not to succeed or shine too brightly via my music and talents so that I would not seem too special. Maybe, just maybe they would love me.

(Again, this is only my perception of what another thought of me.) Yet, when it came to the highest good, from my perspective, asking or "telling" my immediate family it was inexcusable to just disappear and let the daughter go through all of this.   But then SHOW UP at the hospital or nursing home or, memorial. I was pretty raw and tired by then. Little did I know they would disappear again after dad died, when mom had to come live with me.

Finding myself on the black sheep "drama queen" list, and even wanting to relocate to another part of the country and disappear. WOW! When all I really was doing and saying was: "Check in and at least tell our parents, "Thank you for bringing me into the world so I could have this life." Maybe see if they are still alive! I know I must forgive or I remain the one locked in the pain. But this message is about lifting fog. Facing it takes huge courage!

All the while, a little concerned that my own healing brain would be way off. The brain that often could tip me over, take my vision with 3-5 day migraines, multi-fire into wacky seizure-type guck. Was I actually just becoming an egotistical, self-righteous jerk or was I becoming MORE authentic to what is important in this life, aka busting through and lifting the fog and waking up?

So back to horse shit.   That happens to be one of my dad's favorite expressions. I say *happens* because it would not surprise me at all if he is standing around with my grampas, uncles and bestie buddies ... and they are telling stories. Who says there are no swear words in heaven? After all, we made up what a swear word is! We have made up everything here on earth that we call life's perspective – belief - and handed it down generation after generation.

So, as I left the last chapter, still in a thick fog from dad dying, a few days later, I decided to go outside onto my farm. There, I found *another* thick fog. SMOKE. This writing and dad's death happened August 2018. Our WILD FIRE months. Our state and several others were in horrific conditions. Mother Nature was like anger out of control.

My lungs were burning, as I tried to decide if I could go rake and scoop horse poop or not! It wasn't necessary but I felt I had to do some farm work to help my brain work through my grief. Much like dad would do.

Smoke takes oxygen out of the air. Out of us! So when you already have a foggy head, this isn't really the wisest thing to do. But, I went out and raked/scooped horse poop anyway. While raking, scooping, wheel-barrowing the loads to my plants – I reflected on more of the past few months.

Simultaneously, during this journey, searching for insights to help me process dad's pain and death – I happened on to the Ester and Jerry Hicks "Abraham" writings. Channeled insights.   If you are new to this type of information you too might quickly quote my father and proclaim: "HORSE SHIT!" To some, the idea of channeled entities is way too oobie doobie to even consider. But I decided to listen, read, digest and see for myself if my soul agreed. Their talks are a great deal about the law of attraction and the path of least resistance.

During this reflecting – I looked at all of my injuries. My folks, family, love, ending relationships and shifting relationships. I was aware of poverty consciousness. My innate desire to learn 'n grow and be my optimum self. All in the thought that I would get it - When The Fog Lifts. Then, I found myself asking, "So what's really up? Is it my conditions or belief system? Why do I fade in and out of holding onto abundance and worthiness beliefs? Can you hear me dad? Do we really die? Is there a thin veil between death and life?

So here is the profound *scoop from poop*:

As I worked and began feeling ill from the smoke, I watched a bunch of emotions come through. Twice, out of the blue, I busted over and cried hard about dad. Got angry at family. Laughed at funnies that dad gave to me. Smiled with honor, to be the one who led a white horse out at his "life celebration" carrying his cowboy hat, coats and boots. Thank you, Bob! Then, on my last load of poop, I thought about how much I have worried. How much I tried to be accepted by family, by portraying the dummy or poor or good Samaritan or good daughter, sister, aunt, niece, cousin, friend.

I am not kidding! This all happened scoopin' poop! Pushing the full, tippy wheelbarrow out of the field, suddenly I saw dad's face. Clear as a bell. I saw him as if he scanned all those thoughts I had just had and profoundly entered my melon and through the thin veil said loudly, "HORSE SHIT, Sis!" I stopped. "What?" I heard it again: "Horse Shiiiit!"

Oh my gosh! I laughed with shock. In a flash I saw: This is my life. Not the folk in the church. Not the hungry. Not the music business. Not my family. Not those I call friends. Not the neighbors. Not my daughter's. Not any male person that I have shared love with. My life. Let me tell you, if this bites your buttocks - it is pretty dang weird!

The rubber Gumby in me, was so worried about what others thought. How I appeared. If I said or did the right thing to appease, be approved. And when I did speak up, I felt nuts. Like I deserved to be punished.   And here ... in my grief, and a wheel barrow full of horse poop, here comes my daddy with his country boy wisdom through the thin veil exclaiming: it is all HORSE SHIT! Holy moly! That wasn't his only expression, but that was the one for this chapter!

Best I can figure, thus far in my fog lifting, brain-injured interesting experiences – this isn't about not being kind. Not about becoming an opinionated poop head, but about becoming more authentic. Lifting the fog of masks that we wear, hoping that folks will love us. Admire or approve of us.

Just live. Just be. Seek your bliss. Don't harm for your own gain or ego-feast. Death will come calling soon enough. Live! But don't limit your experiences and expressions of life in Fear Of Good. Or Fear Of God. Instead, shovel some of those limiting horse shit thoughts into a big wheelbarrow and go dump it somewhere to rot! Far away! Then, use that foggy compost as insights to fertilize your NEW life. New direction. Give yourself full permission to start again, honor the fog that got you to that place, as school. Then, lift and replace that F.O.G. With: FANTASTIC! OUTRAGEOUS! GOOD! aka healthy F.O.G!

What I learned from being with dad for his exit from earth, was that I WAS in the present, actually. I WAS completely aware. Anger, fear, sorrow, joy, peace, repeat. I wore it all. I don't recommend it as a steady diet, but I WAS there. I was awake.

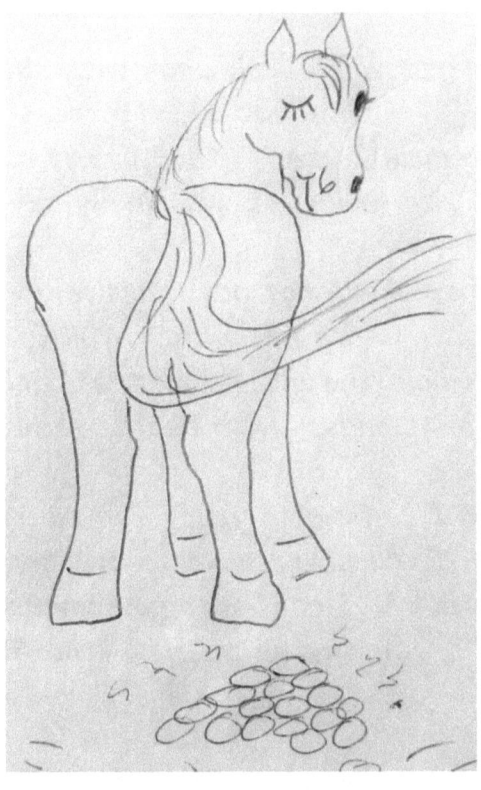

So, is it Horse shit? Or truth?
Answer: Your choice. Your journey. Your life!

Hope this brought a smidgin' or ... Texas-size, shit-load of HOPE as you travel along your path.

If I can blame you - for my pains -
I will never have to own them,
But if I can - let go somehow -
I will find, in my life - the GEM.

A diamond in the rough, polished by time -
will glisten and shine through the world,
because I finally woke myself up -
to a new direction - for this girl.

Never will I look back with shame -
with doubt or bitterness,
because I see - that life is school -
So to life ... I will finally say YES!

I will not go – passively -
into life - NO MORE.
I will hold the ground of trust and truth -
this Lioness, with heart, shall roar.

If I can blame you - for my pains -
I will never have to own them,
But if I can - let go somehow -
I will, find in my life- the GEM.

Chapter 35 – TRAIN BRAIN

With fingers on the keys, I thought this oddity would be worth sharing. We have bloomin' genius, and then - we have just plain *weird*!

One of the peculiar side effects from bonking my head so many times, (could happen with just one) is the pressure that floats around with me that can be pretty severe. Not just migraines. I have had times where I sit at a table and literally lay my head on the table. Or get up in the morning and barely can hold my melon up on my shoulders. Yet, there has never been severity enough to drain the brain. So you live with it, get moving, and hopefully get the spinal fluid flowing throughout the body.

So this train brain thangy. It, I believe, could have made me some great warrior or tracking guide in a past life! "What the heck?" You say!

Beginning with the first hit, I had this weird ability, if you will, to hear in the base of my skull, the low ohms of a train. Now at first, I thought I was totally nuts. I don't mean, the train coming through, just a mile away- I mean, I could hear these low base ohms, "ohm, ohm, ohm" like a kid's bass speakers, yet could not hear it out the window. Only, when I laid down. At one point, I think I even told my daughter's daddy that I believed I could hear electricity in the walls! Yah, okay, that does sound pretty weird!

Of course that got a pretty good "Yes dear, that's nice... now go back to sleep, Laurie."

The wacky thing is, the train was NOT down the road a mile or two. I tried to sleep. Try sleeping with brain injury and with this weird ohmy thingy in your brain! Ha! Right!

I would lay there and feel/hear this sound in the bass of my skull. Ironically, by the time the train passed through our dinky valley, I never put it together, until one night. I awoke. It was 1:00 AM. "Ohm, ohm, ohm" I got up, opened the window. NOTHING. The stillness of the perfect country night. Not even the wind. Went back to bed. Laid there. The split second I laid my head back down, the ohm returned. Only, we aren't talking the meditative relaxing Zen OHM that transcends us to a new level of being. HELL NO! This is aggravating! Keeping me awake!

I laid there. And laid there. And guess what? 1:20, the train whistle blew, right down the hill in our valley! I sat up, I got it! I could hear the ohm at least 20 minutes away! Now, no one else could hear it. Daughter, her dad. Nope. Just me.

Do I feel magically gifted and special because of my train brain? Not! But, because this whole book is about symptoms, journey, condition and healing from the FOG of brain injury... I thought I would share this. That pressure in my skull must push on something in my nerves, that makes this happen. There are nights the train brain does not exist. If I have taken an anti-inflammatory, or Gabapentin, sometimes I am just finally out and cannot hear it. But if I have had pressure all day long, where my walking, balance, thinking was taxed, this could easily be my experience, come night time. Weird huh? Now can you imagine what happens when a kid with a bad-ass bass speaker pulls up beside me? Grrrrr! 'Nuff said!

When fog is thick, too much noise can make me feel so off-balance. Life beyond the door and gate of my farm is FULL of white noise and can be overwhelming. What can you do? When I would drive my pickup - that had a bad muffler or rode in a diesel truck, I would hear that low "Ohm Ohm" for an hour or so, once I would get out of the vehicle. Try telling this to a neurologist!

This writing is just to say, we have to deal with a lot of weird things once our brain has been upset. Pressure is a doozy! Trying to explain this stuff to those around you, is not easy and gets old. So, sharing here, in one fell swoop, well, feels kinda good! After-all, this book was written for me to get this stuff OUT of my brain - in hopes to bring HOPE from inside the "healing" brain-injured brain ... TO YOU! Hey that sounds like a riddle!

One more wacky tidbit.

Pressure. Pressure has one more way of messin' with the head, big time. This is one more *unexplainable* thingy that I get to deal with. This, I *did* tell my neurologist. He did not have any come back. Only to say that I am an *unusual* case, with so many hits! Wee, unusual me!

So here it is: "Hey, Laurie, let's go get Subway for sandwiches!" Cool! Off we go. We arrive. We open the Subway door. Step inside and ...WHAMMO! The base of my skull instantly fills with major pressure like there is no blood flow. I feel like someone is pushing down hard on my head, compressing my spine. I usually have to grab something and wait it out. I do not know how many times I thought I was going to pass out. Sometimes beginning to see black. It's hard to look cool like this!

This one symptom is really freaky. Here is my thunkin' on this weird thing: I think it is... small, enclosed, air-conditioned buildings. My brain has to adjust to the pressure. Train brain and Subway! Yahooosky! Aren't I special!

So, if you need to know if the train is coming, I can lay down on the ground and letcha know for about 20 minutes ahead. And, if you see a chickie getting fainty while getting Subway - you will know why. Weeee!

Train brain go away
don't come back another day
don't like the Ohms that keeps me awake
I'm not a scout for goodness sake!

And holy schmoly give me a break
I like the sandwich that a Subway can make
But hate the ik when I walk through the door
nearly passing out, NO MORE. NO MORE!
LLL

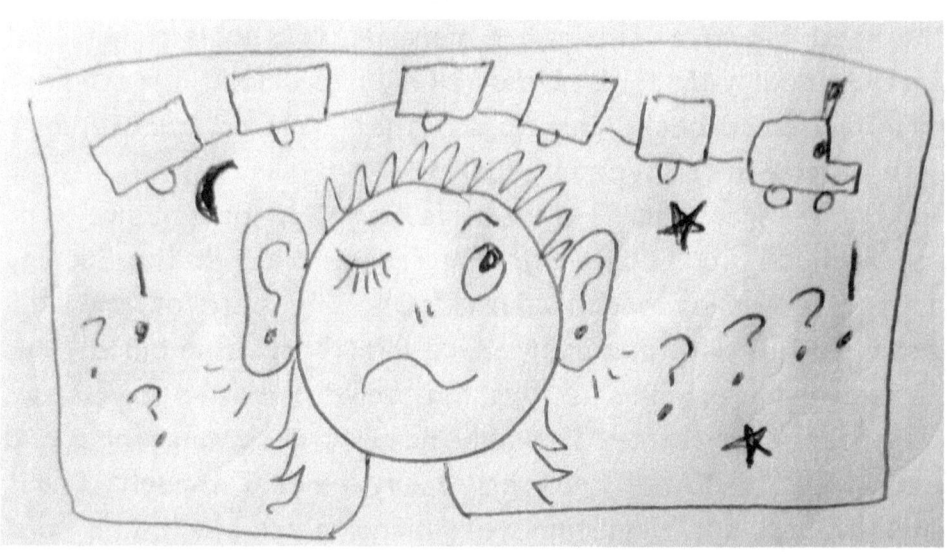

Chapter 36 – Now and Zen

I always wanted to write an entire book with that chapter title. **Now and Zen.** The word Zen is everywhere. It means you are being *mindful* of your *awareness*. **Present**. As I have already written about.   Often Zen is obtained through meditation.   (Funny, the first typing said, Medication!) Obviously, you cannot be meditating and driving - when you need your calm. Try telling the officer, "I was Zenning out!" But *being present* can keep you safe. It is pretty dang hard to find your Zen, when you are deep in fog. Okay fingers let's do this:

I have been given wonderful windows of clear thinking and mostly clear typing in order to go back in time to go through notes, recall, and try to let you know that when the fog moves in, try not to panic. But I would not be completely authentic if I did not tell you, that each time the fog moved in, I never knew for sure, if this one was going to stay. If this one was the pressure in my brain that would take me to my next MRI and find my death sentence. Which also is part of the journey. Sounds dramatic. Trust me, when time passes but symptoms remain, you begin to wonder.

I wanted to include some DAY IN THE FOG moments. I found this short typing that was written Spring 2017: *The past few mornings, I have noticed how thick my head has been. Standing up, my motor skills in my legs, knees, feet are slower and balance off. My feet rock left and right. My eyesight seems off. Ringing in my ears is extra loud. Walking* to the barn to care for my miniature horses and chickens, is about all I can do to get down there and back. I want to cry. But will that help? No. Already enough pressure in my skull.

I am not saying this to dampen this experience, sharing with you.   It is just reality that words are just that.   The experience of no control over balance, time, pain, motor skills, memory. We have to find some grace or- doubt and the damn blues - will want to find us.   Now and Zen?

All I can say in this place, this heart... is: I understand you. I understand your fear. Your questions. Your challenges. Mine might be on a minor scale compared to yours. But I have one foot on each side most of the time, where I am almost unstoppable and want to heal the world, and the other foot on, oops, bad balance today - slow down. "What was I just doing? What is in my hand? Did I leave the tub running, wood stove door open, burner on, pay the bills, turn off the car? Please don't rush me!

Or, should I answer the phone? How long can I tolerate the phone?   What if mom's crippling Osteo is so bad she is suffering massively today and talks about it? Can I handle hearing all about that, all day, today? Can I hear her moan with pain that I cannot fix?

By the time this book hits the public, I know these questions might not even be mine to ask. My beloved dad left us gals here August 2018, making me mom's sudden sole caregiver. As far as knowing about tomorrow, well, plenty of stress could be ahead. So finding my NOW and Zen, I have to take deep breaths.   Go out and listen to the birds. Play with my dog. Play in dirt. Grow things. Life happens.

In a world with so many less fortunate than me, shame on me for worrying about my own condition.   Wait... No. That is not true. We each have to find some ways to check in with our own needs. Our own health. Not just concentrate and focus on another. **You caregivers and loved-ones reading this, you might want to read that again. I just did!**

Our Zen. Our peace of mind. *Critical.*

The latest findings is not only meditation, and the GO WITHIN, but also the social time. The heart to heart we get when we connect with another. Out of the home, the phone. Somehow, remembering there is life out there. Isolation can be dangerous. There is a balance to this whole NOW and ZEN.

Oh I wish I could leave the first typings on some of this stuff. I often speak like Yoda and get a sentence backward. So though you cannot see it, I have had to go through with my pal, spell check, and untie many sentences and put them into some sense of order. Funny. Frustrating. But, in the end, my fingers and I did our best!

I will cool it today. It has taken quite a lot to type this. It is an off day. Foggy. Having to be quiet. Careful. Drink water. Rest.

I'll leave us with this: We don't know which experience might lift fog. It might actually come in a package quite dramatic. Death is often a fog maker and fog lifter - because it ultimately is about love, connection and making life count. Embracing this fog is powerful for soul growth.

Your time, your energy is PRECIOUS. It is okay when you are trying to find the NOW and ZEN combo, to use discernment of others energies around you. Discernment about committing your time. Recognizing that selfish and self-love are TWO different things, but sometimes they have to actually work together for you to take care of YOU! Healing and becoming whole requires self-love.

I dare ya to give yourself a big hug. I double-dare ya to look at yourself in the mirror and say, **"Hey there selfie, I love you!"** If you do, your soul might just whisper back, "THANK YOU, it's about time!"

Chapter 37 – The Blankety Blank

Now I'll just bet that you think I am going to apologize for my swear words, in the previous chapters. Right? Well. Not quite. Since I did not have any clue how to share my journey in text, I have pretty much left this whole book up to writing itself through my fingers, patience, and trying to capture the whole enchilada and make sense. Ha!

Knowing this book is also based on 20 hits or so, over 10 years, drawing off of notes, talking to others about what they recall me acting like, and what I have retained, apparently in order to share. This has been quite a project. So much easier to grow food in dirt and harvest it! Except for the weeding, which is like the hours editing... eeewww iiiik!

What I haven't mentioned much in regards to TBI, post-concussion, stroke, dementia and all the areas that effect the brain is the one that takes the w o r_s aw_y. The simpl_ sto_y that starts out, um, eas_ and slow_y goes bl_ _ _. And there it is. The Blankety Blank. Your radio gets shut off. Dead air space. The void. The empty. You wait. You struggle. You cannot remember that you had a word, a story, a punchline, or you already told/said - it!

Here - I must say, I do not feel alone. Watching dad's Dementia arrive, mom's over-taxed and stressed out brain, the many medicines she has taken for Osteoarthritis, my long-time friend's years of over-medication addiction due to ailments, even my daughter forgetting that we had just visited, due to her busy life. Another friend's concussion, searching for words, repeating stories, and so many others - blank. No memory. No word recall. Some, the blankety blank is advanced. Some, just beginning to show its blankety blank face. Do you know this blank? Most do. Head trauma can include a lot of blank.

Sometimes, I have thought the blank came to us for reasons that are fixable.   Like improving poor listening skills instead of pretending to be present, but, not really.   Or assuming we will see each other again, so just have a surface visit, instead of quality time.   No doubt, life is full. Trying to fit in one more visit or conversation might be the scale tipper. But – we are doing our best.   I think the fact that we keep trying to show up and engage with others says a lot!

I have mentioned this a bit already - about making time together count. Sometimes, you just can't when you are in the injured mode. The fog. Your brain just shuts down. Perhaps over-saturated brains, trying to keep up with family, friends, work, household, taxes, holidays, Dr. appointments, etc... maybe we fry some wires. Maybe it is burn-out. Maybe the burn-out brings the fog. The fog brings the injury.   We develop survival skills to help with memory and the blank. The doctor's visit.   The grocery shopping nightmare.   The errands, needs, that are put upon our lives.

The blank space that shows up when you need your recall, can leave you both mad and sad at the idea that it is getting worse. Even scared. Of course now that science is learning that multiple head injuries can leave a very blank outcome – I have had to deal with this reality, but it has made me cherish NOW even more.

Maybe, this knowing, boosts my ornery willpower that says NO!   I will not lose my brain! If I do, I am installing a clap-on, clap-off, lamp turn-on device! Or beeping key finder. Not sure how to install it yet, but dang it, I won't go into the blankety blank without a fight!

I will take my vitamins. My herbs. My hydration. My exercise. My continued learning to stay activated. My dad's face is burned in my memories. I see his smiles pre-brain injury. Then I see the misery. I see the blank. The glaze. So painful. I see his life's journey of many hits, stroke, many years prior of drinking, (dry since 1980), chemical poisoning work injury, and, 84-years-old, when he finally was released from the pain.

What I hold as important, is how, before the Dementia took hold strongly, when dad would talk to you, he did not just rattle off words to hear himself speak. He had something to say. Something to ask. For the most part, would do his darndest to hear you. THAT, is quality. Sure, he could gripe with the best of them, and swear – in pissed-off sentences - that you did not know could exist. But in his soul – his communicating soul – he cared what you said. Where you had been. He WAS present. That is a worthy goal for me. Not so far thinking in front. Not dwelling or living in the past. But trying to take in the present/now. Slower, with joy.

If you find in this book that I repeat, well, you will never know if it was brain-blank farts that I forgot I typed-OR that intuitively, I shared again, to make a point. With dementia and brain injuries, repeating is a very common part. It can drive you nuts! The caregiver can finish the stories. And at times, hard not to. Professional caregivers are trained to: "enter client's world" not force them - back out to yours. The goal of this writing is expressing what it is like to be inside the fog, trapped, and trying to find ways to lift it - to a better quality of life.

As for the blankety blank space - suggestions to caregivers who want to finish our sentences, take in a deep breath. Go gentle. Lean in. Soften. If you must, for your sanity, even hum. Maybe softly help us remember. But please, do not add to our pain, and make us feel like an idiot, blarring out "YOU just said that!" We have enough going on.   And, in return, I will try to do the same. If we fail, we can always say, "I AM SORRY." We cannot FIX this blankety blank part! But we can use it to listen, learn, lean in, and love. Honestly, a little "good job" kudos, as I gave to my dad, is a pretty damn nice thing to hear, when you are getting deeper in fog.

I remember telling dear Michael, as we prepared to sell a few plants the Spring 2017, to support the farm, (also writing about the blankness): "I know that this book is coming through right now in its own timing. Whether or not I can do such writing a year from now – I don't know. So I really give thanks for NOW."   Michael was gracious and said, "You will. I know you will. I have faith in you, Lil One." (His nickname for me.)

Oh you dirty son-of-a-gun,
I had the word - but it done run -
right out of my brain and off my face,
that Blankety blank - injured space.

Come back, come back,
name, face and words -
where did you go?
This is absurd!

Will you return?
Am I stuck in this pain?
Come on FOG lift...
this blankety blank brain.
LLL

Chapter 38 – Disabled and dis-ability

Okay I said in the beginning, that I wasn't going to write this book from my dented noggin' with fancy schmancy cut and pasting from Google-world. Well, it was on my heart to include a chapter about disability. I referred to this in the beginning of this book, when I went to see the brain specialist, Dr. J., for HOPE - not to be assessed for *disability*.

So with full intention of writing, I opened my laptop to the blank page that was here just before my fingers agreed to try to communicate with my head and fill it with these words. Here we go: Wait... wait... and then, blank. Come on, Laurie! Look at the top of the page. Disability. Disabled. Remember? What do I really feel and want to say about this? It was there before I hit the power button and turned on my laptop. What the heck! Where did my writing thoughts go? Daggum it!

This is kinda like, "Hey, guess what happened to me today?" But before you can get out your story someone tells you theirs. Then it is... aaah, BLANK! Nothin. Zippo. Where do thoughts go? For the brain-injured it might go like this: Who took my keys? Why can't I make eye contact today? Why do I feel like crying? Who left the burner on? Why are my knees buckling when I walk? What is the wave of dizzy that keeps wanting to topple me over? What day is it? Did I forget an appointment or somebody? Who flooded the bathroom with the bathtub? What is burning? What pant's zipper? Why can't I sleep? Same clothes three days later? Really? When will the ringing ears stop? When will the vice be taken off my skull? Why do I have days when I hate brushing my hair cuz it hurts and want to shave my head? Whew. Dramatic? Remember, I am writing this as a voice. For all of us.

Wait, there's more. Why do I get anxious about travel and making plans? Why do I have days I would like to not wake up? Why do I feel like a hypochondriac? When will the Ginko Biloba, Taurine and Fish oil kick in? Why can others handle loud noises, coffee shops, dishes clanging, grocery stores, but I cringe? Who forgot to eat and let her blood sugar plummet? Who forgot to pay the power bill cuz she lost it? Why do piles of papers over-whelm me? Who left her list at home and cannot remember one thing to buy? Who forgot why she walked outside? Who forgot what she did yesterday with her often next-morning amnesia? Who fears one day she might forget the most important people in her life? Including me.

But then... the fog would lift... when my head has a clear day or half day, and hot doggies... I nearly float with gratitude and can't understand why healthy people aren't floating all the time! And ... who is writing this book? How can this be possible? When just a few hits ago, all my words were backward when I tried to write.

So today – upon starting to write this subject, blanket-y blank BLANK arrived... no words about disability. Lost my train of thought.

Can you see what I am trying to share here, in the moment? So, to re-inspire my brain, I thought I would go grab Uncle Webster's description of disability. Yes, okay, a teeny weeny cut and paste. Uncle Web says: **Disability**

1. **lack of adequate power, strength, or physical or mental ability; incapacity. 2. a physical or mental handicap, especially one that prevents a person from**

living a full, normal life or from holding a gainful job.

In reality, the list above of forget-me-a-lots... can apply to many people, with or without brain injury. As I said in the beginning, any incident that causes big changes, loss, birth, moving, divorce, IRS, jobs - can bring FOG. And if fear is attached the fog might get thicker. The sooner we address the fear, not let it win, the fog can begin to lift.

Literal "lost in fog" can cause horrible accidents. My family knows this well. I will never forget attending our beloved cousin Rick's memorial service. Simply driving to work in the early morning, when hit head-on by another vehicle, killing our beautiful cousin and his friend/co-worker.

Could this have been prevented? In the cosmic plan? Is this how life works? They were just loyally going to work. There death brought many people together. Touched many lives. Reminded us that life should be treasured and live now. Hug more. Not let fear ruin our lives. Having FAITH OF GOOD instead of FEAR OF GOOD. Once we understand even this much about F.O.G. We can shift.

I do not ever proclaim to know what is a meant to be and what is an accident. I just know mental fog can be a big sign that our lives are off balance. Please take caution to take extra care while in the fog.

A fog that has had me sorting through if it is fear of good or embarrassed, surrender or quitting, has been the subject of disability. Talking to several people, once again it came up that I should consider filing with Social Security for SSI. My quick reply was "I have not worked enough in my life, as a stay-home mom for over 18 years. I do not deserve that which I did not pay in to." But a friend told me lovingly, something that I had not thought of. He said, "Think of this as temporary help, to heal." Wow. My focus was - if I try for disability, that is, if you can get through the 6 months to a year of waiting, denials, appeals, court, doctor, visits etc... (like TBI isn't enough to deal with) and having to convince others of this when you don't want to focus on the negative. Should I?

What does this mean? Is my faith to heal not strong enough? What will happen to my pride? And, will I surrender and declare I am disabled? Unable? I can grow flowers and produce at my own pace. Will others call me a user of the system? Fake? A wimp? Gosh, for a moment I felt like 7 years old, right there. My brother and some classmates calling me a wimp because I was pulled out of recess for two years, do to a cartilage issue with my knees, that could have left me crippled. All that worry again of what others will think and what I will think! Pee-yewsky! Worry... What a waste.

I cannot tell you what grief these thoughts brought through my system. I assume that I am not alone. I've had days where I feel so blessed and able - that there is no way I should even be on this page, pondering disability. Then days at the grocery store, where the floor tipped and sent me to the left, where, luckily my daughter was standing, there to stop me. My goofy balance. Just dealing with everyday life.

To apply or not to apply for disability. The jury stayed out debating. My belief remained that a song, a story, this book, something of my life experience was moving to the front of my soul path and wa-la, income. No problem. No worries of losing my house. No worries of buying feed for my critters or myself. Seriously tired of the bank notifying me that my balance is $4.68! ENOUGH!

All I can think of, and choose to believe, is that everything I go through, I have somehow set up as soul school to learn from. So, about 32 and a ½ % of me considered going through the whole "experience" of filing for disability with no attachment.

Somehow, about 2 weeks after I decided this, I found

a law firm that could do the proper filing out of Tennessee. Seemed very, very weird to me that they could file this stuff in my state. Many calls to them first - assured me: no disability, no debt owed. They would take up to 30% first payment. So I said okay. Let's try.

Suddenly I was filling out papers and getting contract agreements in the mail. Social Security letters preparing me for the next few months. I kept taking deep breaths trying not to let FEAR win. Fear of what? I focused on the fact I would have to eventually sit in front of a hearing most likely, and state my case. Thinking, well, this is school of life to share with others, so if nothing more than whomever comes in contact with me and my case, will be exposed to this journey of TBI and my message: LIFE IS A GIFT.

Considering I did not know what I was going to say in this chapter, and my fingers brain-farted and just sat on the computer keys... I think I did alright.

I filed. I waited. But then, Laurie or Laurie's pride showed up.

One morning I awoke full of MOXY. The I CAN DO IT. I am NOT DISABLED. I will write this daggum book. Write my songs. Grow my foods. Support myself! Find a way to make moola and I will not be locked into income limitation via Washington state watching over me.

When I learned the amount of disability, like $720 a month for S.S.I, I was told that if I made money, at all, I had to report it. But got to keep the first $60 bucks. Yay. But then whatever I reported, say, $200 for garage sale, should I be that honest, the state would reduce my check to $580. I report $800 for auto sale or something, that month is zero. How about that? Sign up and be limited.

For someone who is unable to do anything to make income - this is money. It will help. But be prepared for a long journey. For me, I just could not do it. I called the attorneys and said no. They actually debated with me, looking at my brain injury record. Ha! I 'spose they see Dementia in the future. And possibly present, in the fact that I was calling to cancel filing!

I even had the cool neurologist and my primary doctor ready and willing to fill out all the papers on my behalf. Dumb on me? Ashamed? NO. I had to think and pray about this a lot before I typed it. I don't think so. I just needed the road traveled to come to my own awakening that I AM lifting fog and this journey will make sense.

I do want to say to you, what I learned from this: if you do opt to go this direction, beforehand, hold your head up high. If you have records at doctors or need fresh ones, get to your family doc. Get a CT scan, fresh blood work, describe in detail, your symptoms. Get to a neurologist if you possibly can.

Do not be ashamed or embarrassed to ask for financial help. If a doctor strapped on yours or my head for a day, a few hours, they would freak. They could NOT do their job. They could not bring home the hefty paycheck that they receive, because WE needed them.

It is all tied together. When we see this, we have no NEED to be embarrassed. Honestly, I have had at least 4 appointments with neurologists that basically sat in a chair, nodded, agreed, and I did all the work. I thought damn, easy money. In fact, at one point, I remember one of them telling me about them, and at one point in their over-lit, stuffy exam room, I thought, "I wonder just how much this person is earning this moment, as he/she looks at me, and is telling me about their stuff!"

Filing for disability it isn't a sweet, take-advantage, user ride! It takes some big balls to have the courage to apply in the first place! Especially with the horrible tests they put you through. Pay no attention to the author. If you need it, be brave. DO it.

Chapter 39 - It's All In Your Head!

I certainly did not write this book as a bitching/venting opportunity. Though, some of the chapters may sound that way. Rather, it has been a way for me, myself and I - to cut through fog. (at least I am not alone with all 3 of me.) Testing your humor here! This has been my way to seek a higher way of looking at rough stuff in my life's journey. I figured if I dare share, maybe my wacky story would bring a little light beaming through another's fog. Sometimes, just shifting thoughts - lifts the fog.

As I have mentioned before, we do not have to choose to believe in purpose, miracles, meant-to-be'ums.! In fact, if you are wired scientifically, it is very difficult for the mind to comprehend that - which cannot be proven.

We ARE the miracles. Think about it. If ya can. Our brain, heart, skin, organs and breath are proof of that. We could have been born a rock. A cold rock. Just hangin' out with other cold rocks. Oh wait, I think we do have a few humans in society that kinda chill together lacking warmth, but, they started out warm, life just turned them cold.

I do have one pet peeve. I have mentioned a time or three about visits to doctors, where you walk in and walk back out and wonder why you went - and what the heck they do. I know I always find out how much I weigh and how my oxygen level and blood pressure are. That is cool. Tells me I am still pumpin!

The brain doctors. Some seem like Gods, when you

finally get the appointment. Months out. Why is that? The assumption by the *laymen brain-injured person* is that when it says neurologist, you naturally assume they are up on concussions. BRRRRAIN problems. I appreciate that they got their degree that hangs on the wall, that says neurologist... I just have yet to figure out how my brain fits in with their service.

Two appointments I have gone to, I simply sat face to face – talking. Like, over coffee. But there was no coffee. There was crappy florescent lights. Small room. Had to shut one light out. Nice magazine. No balance tests. No hand-writing abilities. No math. No spelling. Oh, wait, I think a finger went in front of my nose to track back and forth. And, oh yes, a thumpy thing went on my knees to check reactions.

Now if this is a return visit, maybe they have ordered an MRI or CT scan. Doubtful though. That will be after this appointment if you prove insurance worthy of the scans. Perhaps YOU will have to ballsy-up and ask for one!

During the appointment - you do your best. You know you are forgetting stuff. You may or may not have made a list to be your poor brain's memory under pressure of those overly-lit dinky exam rooms and rushed time. You may or may not have brought someone with you to remember with and for you! Pressure is on. Will this be the answer? Will this appointment be the miracle fog-lifter? At least, when ya have a cavity, dentist grinds, fills, fixes. Brain, notta.

Perhaps, like me, tired of the journey, with recent days of tipping over, heavy head, walking like a duck, knees buckling, 2-day headache, unable to sleep, and loss of sight for an hour due to a migraine. Oh, and trying to fight off the darkness, one just isn't impressed with a doc appointment.

When you do get to the appointment, your doctor should be taking notes, opening files of labs or any recent MRI or CT. This is the moment of hopeful clarity. This is the clincher that the majority of TBI, post-concussion brains hear: "Well, your MRI or CT looks fine. No tumors. No bleeding. Nothing. "Of course, we did not use CONTRAST in your veins on the last MRI, at your request, so if there was something, that might have shown it". Otherwise your brain looks good!

You look over their shoulder and maybe see this weirdness:

Exam	Date:		03/14/2018
CT	HEAD	W/O	CONTRAST
Clinical:	Headaches,	amnesia,	ataxia.
Comparison:	Head	CT from	3/29/2011.

Procedure: Standard Head CT imaging performed without IV contrast. CT was performed with dose optimization techniques to lessen patient radiation   exposure.

Findings: No midline shift, mass effect, or extra-axial fluid collection. No hydrocephalus. The basilar cisterns are patent. No evidence of acute intracranial hemorrhage or infarct. No cerebral volume loss or focal encephalomalacia. Midline structures and craniocervical junction appear   normal.

Paranasal sinuses and mastoid air cells are clear. No acute skull fracture.

IMPRESSION:

1. Negative noncontrast head CT with no evidence of an acute intracranial   abnormality.

Silence. I think this was my 3rd MRI in 4 years. The 4th finally showed "white marks all over, from trauma."

But this reading and appointment... of course you want to hear that everything looks normal. Of course you do! Right? But why do I feel tears wanting to come out? Why do I want to get the hell out of that overly-lit exam room?

Then your mind starts zipping around with questions. Was I hoping for a tumor? OMGosh! How demented is that? What was I hoping for? Or maybe more realistically showing fluid? Something to explain my heavy, good day/bad day - head.

The time is up, appointment is over and the doctor suggests Ibuprofen and time. Or, a counselor perhaps! Or, massage therapy. (Okay now that one would be nice!)

He/she suggests you take it easy, and see them again in a 6 month to year follow up. No. You did not get any answer. Wait! What did the doctor/specialist just say? Am I fine? Yes, Laurie, your brain looks fine!

This is the nuttiest, craziest experience when you know what you are going through. You know the hell your brain puts you through when no one is looking or even when they are! You know you use to be a different person. Further more, if you drove yourself there, can you drive home?

You know your emotions are upside down. You know you do not sleep. You know you lost your sight the day before, followed by a migraine that almost made you vomit! You know YOUR life has changed. And deep down, you know you do NOT want a tumor found. But that little bit of WHY ... is there.

At the end of the appointment, basically you walk out as you walked in, pick up some papers and leave the office not healed. But, if the appointment did not bring a little bit of comfort, the worse might happen: you might conclude your worst fear: **It's all in your head!** That somehow, someway, you made this up. You became a hypochondriac and you actually healed a long time ago, but just didn't get the memo!

REALITY: Damn straight... it is all in your **head.** YES. You were injured. YES. You have been changed. For how long will

265

you be this way? No one knows. Is this the new you? If so, what will you do with the new you? The specialist gave you the scientific, facts right there on the screen: "Your brain looks fine."

Walking to the parking lot: stunned, dazed and confused, no different than you walked in, only with a result of "brain looks fine" running through... the profoundly deep reaction finally might arise: "Shhhhhhhhiiiiiiit!" Or, "Oh poopie kaka" whichever fits your vocabulary style the best. Or, who knows, could be the total opposite. You might take a deep breath in, and say, Praise the Lord! No Tumor!

So why write this chapter: **It's all in your head**?

ABSOLUTELY: IT'S ALL IN YOUR HEAD!
ABSOLUTELY: IT'S ALL IN YOUR HEAD!
ABSOLUTELY: IT'S ALL IN YOUR HEAD!
ABSOLUTELY: IT'S ALL IN YOUR HEAD!

Did you just read that 4 times? Well, that is how many MRI(s) I have had. That is how many CT scans I have had. It is how I have traveled this road in 10 years.

The MRIs and CT scans of the past were a waiting game. Many days passed, to see if you were about to head down a long road, or got a green light that everything was okay. Now days, luckily, it is very fast. One ER CT scan, the tech asked if I had eaten in the past like 8 hours. I answered yes. He said, "Oh, well if we find fluid and need emergency surgery to drain it, we need to know when you ate last." My fogged brain thought: So, if I ate oatmeal for breakfast, you will make me fast before you can save my life from brain swelling?" Ooopsie on me.

There is such a twist of emotions. Round and round. BUT... the truth is, the doctor did not wake up that day ... to ruin *your* day - nor did they erase something from your Xray! They aren't lying. They are actually telling you - that though you are injured, you are not dying. They are ACTUALLY trying to be hopeful!

Now some reading this, may have had a tumor removed that could or would have taken your life. *IT'S ALL IN YOUR HEAD.* But hopefully, and thankfully to surgeons, it was removed and you are healing.

I had absolutely no idea I would write such a chapter. I was literally *finally* drifting off to sleep, exhausted from a migraine the night before, a CT and 2 doc appointments, worried about my folks, minimal sleep, then came the whisper: *"Laurie, get up, turn on the laptop. I have some words for you. Type: It's all in your head. Because the words you are about to type, every belief system you have, every thing you have learned about yourself, love, God, kindness, fog, hate, joy, fear, choices and so on ...* IT'S ALL IN YOUR HEAD.

So I typed. However fingers, I would like to end it with this: I DISAGREE! I don't think it is ALL in my head! I think... some of it... is in my ... **heart**! "Whaaaat?" You might ask, after reading all the heady stuff! Yah. Your heart. Not ALL your head. (Hey I am even shaking my head gently at "my head!) Because, if you believe everything appears as-is, at face-value - you stop *sensing* through life's greatest filter and just go with words and thoughts. That filter is: y*our* feelings. *Your* heart. *Your* intuition.

The idea that the fog of this condition has put you here, right now – reading this - taking in new information. If it asks you to get quiet and let your heart speak, listen to it! If it gets you feeling first, then thinking, tada! YOU DID IT! Just busted up and lifted some fog. BRAVO!

The heart. Then the head. No matter *what* happened to the head. If it can be a blessing in OPENING THE HEART to life - in its fullness and depth. Crazy huh? Right there in front of us!

I think I should turn this into the WHO'S ON FIRST?

WHAT'S ON SECOND! The chicken or the egg joke. Head? Heart? Head is the computer. Heart is the filter and power source!

So the question a chewin' on my buttocks is egging me on to ask:
In looking at your journey to NOW, *which* has led you to this moment, reading these words? *Your brain* has certainly helped you comprehend this singing farmer's jargon. MY OH MY! But what led you to this interest or path that got you to read about one woman's journey through multiple concussions and messages of hope? Do you think *your heart* led you here? Mine certainly did.

In all the things I would rather be doing... the biggest teaser of all and devoted commitment to finish this book, has been that I worked hard through winter, using the cold weather to write, knowing the moment the sun and warmth returned to my farm, ta heck with editing! Sun up til sun down, dirt will call. And, I had made a promise to my dad, before he died, that I would share my story. Our story.

Well I typed all winter, but sure enough, Spring arrived and I am actually typing these words with dirty fingernails! YUP YUP YUP. While farming has been more for my body, mind, spirit... and barely made me a plug nickle over the years, being able to grow foods, donate to food banks, and share flowers... has been amazing!

So back to head *or* heart:
Now, to fulfill my promise to myself, the birdies are singing, my bib overalls and work boots are waiting. The tractor sits on the battery charger saying, "Come ye hither lil farm gal, fire me up and let's git'r done!"

So the only way I can do this book during farming season, so you can read it... I must type by the light of the moon, roll into bed with a over-worked back, get up and hit'r in the morning – then out I go! Or wait for the rains.

But guess what? My heart is still leading. Because when I think about you reading this, you being in the fog. Me being SO GRATEFUL to even remember how to start my tractor – and bend over to tend to plants or type ... and if if if... my words bring just a little sparkle of hope to you - then my heart is dancin' a jig in the dirt!

Yup! Damn straight! My mind has had to journey all over the place. From the darkest dark to the beaming light of inspiration, and like the farmer in me, prep soil, plant seeds, tend to them. Harvest. That has been my brain. Getting ready for these long 10 years, to share all of this.

So YOU. What led you here? Your brain? Or, Your heart? If you have no idea what I mean by the heart being the filter, then more than likely, you are brain-oriented. BUT... if you bonked your brain, and you have been in brain-mode all your life, I say there is a pretty good chance that a huge wake up call with your soul agreement just rang your door bell! Sayin', "Hey, brainie... you *think* too much. How's about you *feel* for a change. How's about you get back to the heart-centered life that you were given when ya popped from the womb!"

Okay then, well, *my brain* has been completely scrambled watching all of those words unfold on the screen! Hmm. The next time you hear: "It's all in your head" I wonder if you will remember this yapping by Ye Ol' 20-some hit wonder?

It *is* in your head. Because in reality, we, and only we, can tell our head how we are going to use this experience. Injury and illness show us what we are really made of.

So, if a good friend, should say to you, if you are in the post-hit fog, and trying to find your way out: "YOU ARE NOT YOUR HEAD INJURY," you are aloud to reply, "Today, I AM."

Chapter 40 - Impulsive Spontaneity!

Okay, you will never know how long it took to come up with those two words to describe what I want to share here. Much less, try to spell them! It goes something like this with brain injury. As you go through this fog, trying to cope, heal, adapt... you may have some times that you may experience being impulsive OR spontaneous. This can feel similar when they happen from a drug or alcohol-induced brain. But you quickly find out in some cases, just what shape you are actually in. Sometimes, if there is someone going through this with you, they may have to use some intervention.

Impulsive - basically you go do it without thinking.
Spontaneous - you might say "Sure, why not!" and stretch yourself to have fun.

Impulsive isn't always about having fun. It is can be like a surge: I will do this, damn it, and you will not stop me. Or I MUST get this done. Or I will text, email, call without forethought.

In reality, I have gotten a lot done, being impulsive. I have also started projects and panicked at the OH MY GOSH, what have I done. I cannot finish this! Or I have purchased things, (not often) but just because. Okay, I usually end up taking things back, but I think you know what I mean! Or offered to hold an event because THAT particular day, I was fog-free! I forgot the stress that can accompany an event.

When I say someone might have to be the voice of

reason, in actually trying to protect you, this gets pretty screwy. Because you may find you get angry when someone does this. Like they are trying to control you. Which, depending on each situation, maybe be partially true!

On the flip, those around you may forget what you are going through, or, simply not understand. So, when invitations to say, go to the fair, or a movie, or city, or mall... and you want to try to fit in – this can end in disaster.

I have a few scary things that come to mind:

Once, I went to the movies with my daughter, her beau and lovely cowboy Bob, (who stayed at my home for 6 months, in his 5th wheel with horses). Good movie, but action-packed. I had not been out to one for a long time. When we came out, my brain was really tired. That, and the lighting of the mall, my knees buckled, I could barely walk. Eyes spazzed. Not fun. Embarrassing and scary. They managed to get me out to the truck. I was embarrassed and would have been stuck without them, probably crawling on the floor.

Another movie, same thing, tried to go, too much movement on the screen and I started to fall out of my chair. I had to go wait in the lobby. Dang, I felt bad, family felt bad and it wasted movie money!

The biggest one, so desperately wanting to have fun with my daughter, I knew it was too much, but wanted to go to the fair with her. Normally, I would hold her arm, and I could focus on something to get me through on-coming people and stimuli.

We arrived at the fair during the busiest time. I told her I thought I would be okay for a bit if she wanted to go find her friend and visit awhile. I sat alone on a bench. Then decided maybe I could try to walk the main road through the grounds instead of the barns. (More space, so I thought.)

I had no more than gotten about 1/3 of the way on the main road when my eyes realized hundreds of people were coming at me, passing me on the left, right, crossing in front of me, coming up behind... flags, colors, smells, feet, faces... on and on! I stopped. I began to shake. My heart rate went up. I felt swirly. Knees started to buckle. In a panic I felt like getting on the ground and crawling to a tent. HELP! I didn't think to text my daughter. I went blank. *This* was so terrifying. It was like driving the wrong way on the freeway.

It felt like a quantum moment in time. Like my identity and space were all mixed up. I just stood there shaking, trying not to cry.

Then, in the chaos, of noise, commotion and smells, my brain or an angel sent me a message. It said, "Laurie, look down, about 3 feet in front of you on the ground - and begin to walk. Do not look at faces. Go straight, until you see space and turn into the space. So I did.

I cannot tell you how long I was in that orb, but when I saw feet-less space, I turned left, saw grass and bleachers. Just before my knees buckled, I sat down on the grass and shook. I could not understand what was wrong with me. Why could I not be like a normal person/mom, taking her daughter to the fair? Then, a text came in, "Hey mom, are you okay?" Callie sensed it.

I tell you these embarrassing stories because I am stubborn. I admit that. I have had to miss quite a few things due to injured brain. Had to say no. Cancel. Cut things short. So when the fog would start to lift, there was that fine line of when are you strong enough or not?" Impulsively, I might say "YES, lets go shop at midnight!" Then seriously regret driving in the dark, the bright store lights, and having to get home. Or camping. Or accepting a music gig. So many things. That fine line of time, is, "Are you well enough to do this or are you just trying to please someone else, feel obligated or convince yourself?

I do not have an answer of how to know which is which. If you feel *spontaneous* to go to the movies, I would say, just guessing here, that spontaneous is the healthy version. *Impulsive*, jump in, go do - can have some risks. It is almost that little counting of *common sense*: one one-thousand, two one-thousand... just a pause and deep breath, to check in with yourself or, again, the injured one, and see just HOW BIG this idea is, particularly, if the injury is still fresh. I can't tell ya how many times we took my mom and dad on Sunday drives to start out good and dad rapidly fade. Suddenly dealing with a different guy. Trying to get him home.

We won't know, until we try. Heck, I saw some severely injured folk at the TBI conference I attended, and they seemed like they were handling the environment so much better than me! The carpets, lighting and people was about all I could handle. But some, just smiled and were happy to be there! Perhaps not so sensitive to their surroundings.

Yes I can. No I can't
What was I thinking?
I just woke up to way too much
My safety alarm is blinking.

When can I just do the do
like everyone else around me?
I really try and it is called:
Impulsive Spontaneity.

LLL

Chapter 41 - Nuts!

There are some things very hard to type. Not quite sure how to express. Ha! Imagine that, this deep into the book. But it has to do with looking back after a head injury or any seriously FOGGED-IN time in your life – and wonder what critical decisions you made?

Some of us may easily be looking back pre-concussion and see a pretty good marriage. Decent communication. Romance. Friendship. A purchase. But then came the hit. And suddenly everything was skewed left or right. Nothing ever quite made 100% sense. Ooof, and then, when the fog lifted, the proverbial expression, "How de hell did I get here?" appears!

This is the case for me. Even today, years after divorced from a 16-year marriage, I will have quantum flashes. Perhaps drifting off to sleep, then suddenly wide awake, of wondering what is real! I got up and opened the laptop at 1 AM to write this, remembering special times as a little family. Camping. Singing. Creating. I smile at the memories. But then, a piece of me wants to cry for a moment too.

I have to remember where I was at the time our marriage came to an end. Two minds and hearts no longer on the same playing field. My mind altered, slower and not willing to tolerate some areas my then, husband had become more extreme on. He too was in survival mode with an injured wife. Thinking back - a weird flash returned. Me, sleeping in a closet, following one hit. Yes, a closet.

A pinnacle shift was happening, but I did not know it. I only knew I needed space and our house just was not set up with an extra bedroom. Only my office. So, at night, I slept in the closet of the office. I can't tell you for how long, but I feel it was several weeks. We are talking cot-size foam on a maybe 3' wide board. Yah. Weird. I know. I did mention I hit my head, right? Just keepin' it real, here.

It seemed it was at a point when my intellectual ex-husband was maxed. I would ask a question and NEED a short answer. Yet I would get a long version and perhaps many ways to do one thing.   TOO MUCH OF TOO MUCH with a foggy brain. (I still get exhausted around this type of person.)

Try as I may to explain my needs, what ended up was me feeling dumb. Slow. Shutting down. The intellect amplified my condition. Granted, multi-hitters like me are exhausting to a family. Much less, myself!   To have your wife or mama getting better and joining the human race again and kerpowy - hit again. Back down the black hole.   This is hard to write.

So why did I call this chapter: Ah, NUTS!?   Well, normally that would be the expression for "Ah, shoot I forgot my..." Well, there was a lot of that over a 10-year span. Turn around and forget and forget and ... forget.   "Ah, nuts!" And back I would go, stand in the house and think, "What the heck was I just planning to do or need or have?" None of this is fun. But I am not alone with this experience. Many people forget!

When you forget frequently or wake up in a closet, you begin to wonder, ah, um, NUTS?   But, since this whole book is about taking my goofy brain thumpin' journey and gleaning the good from it, to remove Fear Of Good or Fear Of God, and maybe lift some fog and give hope – well, telling you that I know this nutty road ... is still on track with my intentions.

To look straight into your own deepest fears and totally

decide that fear will not own me or win - wow! Or that you ARE afraid! Wow! Being honest! That is some serious stuff. Even the greatest motivational speakers will say they have a blink or a mountain of doubt. But they pressed on. They have seen what happens when you take challenges and turn them into lessons of growing – and then, turn around and share those lessons with others.

I live my life daily as if it is the last day. Best I can. It makes it a bit hard to plan out too far - living like that. But helps us be more present today! Sometimes it is because I have the knowing that I have hit many times. After each hit, I said that *that* was the LAST ONE. Never in my wildest imagination would have I even whispered, "Hey Laurie, that aint the last one." No way! Hells bells, I am editing in Spring of 2019, and in the simple act of checking a rat trap one night, I moved a pole which hit a steel pole above my head and brought it down and WHOP. Then bounced off my head and hit my arm.

I am NOT listing this one on the whops. I refuse to. Even if it did make my eyes water! I have a very painful spot on the left side of my head. But, at least I told someone! You. Just now! Good girl, Laurie.

Even when I cried with frustration and such sorrow watching my dad disappear more and more daily I tried to glean what I could, from what he was teaching me. His was simple windows of drinking a little coffee, or grinning at his own gas, holding my hand or getting kisses from "one" of his wives. Those precious moments when he did not feel nuts... and knew he was still himself, and alive. Seeing him not plagued by the "gotta do" list as much. But, without "doing" dad was dying. His whole life was a git'r done life. Perhaps that is the most vicious part of Dementia and the brain not working. The desire to do, but the ability to follow through is blank. Gone.

I 'spose this writing is really once again to say, if you are going through the fog right now – whatever it is, or your loved-one, and you are trying to understand - I would have to say that "grace" is seriously needed during these windows. A softening. You are not nuts! Or, THEY are not nuts!

If you wake up a year or two later and look back at the big question, "Did I make the right decision? Well, try to go with the "Everything happens for a reason" angle. Let that hold true that your life, your head, your growing, your fog, it is not a mistake. It IS happening for your highest good. And when you can accept that – fog will lift.

Profound pondering moment:

To get to the fruit
ya may have to go out on a limb.

To get to the meat of a nut,
Ya may have to hit its shell.

Oooh, Bad description, Laurie
Really bad description!
LLL

Chapter 42 - Survival Mode

Since we cannot speed up the healing of the brain and while everyone around us might try to encourage us to rest with: "You will get better" cheer-leading, we the brain know how hard it is on everyone. If we get sad, mad, fogged-in, can't communicate, have to cancel things, get overwhelmed and the rest of the list, it all adds together. All we can do, if we remember, is come back to hope and one day at a time.

Meanwhile, just like if you had the flu and knew that you had to do a whole lot of up-chuckin' to get well, much like patients going through chemotherapy, we have to switch to *survival mode*. We don't know how long things last. We hope today is the worst day. Tomorrow much better. My 5-6 day migraines, I was ready to be put down, like a horse,

I wonder sometimes if those who rarely have any foggy things happen to them, then they get nailed with food poisoning or the flu – if they are capable of understanding that THIS is what many people go through. Not just them. An opportunity to empathize with our world family about suffering? I know once a woman goes through labor, she is never the same as far as wondering about women going through labor. Oh my gosh!   Brain injuries are so vast in symptoms, that the word FOG is the best fit.

Survival mode might go something like this: Where am I? Where did I go? Who is controlling my motor skills? Why don't my words come out? Why is everyone so loud? Why do they talk so much? Why doesn't my hand and pen make words on paper? Why do I tip over? Why are my ears ringing so loudly and never stop? Why do I have another headache?

Why does my face feel numb? Why do I stutter? Why do I fear crowds? Why do I get dizzy with moving objects? Why do I avoid conflict? Or want to argue? Who can I blame? Can this possibly have a meaning? Why do I feel so alone? Why do I feel so depressed? Why do I feel like the world is focused on the wrong meaning of life? Why do I hate malls? Why can't I drive? Why do I feel like a burden?

The list goes on, during survival mode.

There are so many books out there written by neurosurgeons, psychologists, brainyologist specialists, but you, or me, or your loved-one, we IS da brain. Trapped behind the eyes. Between the ears. Deep in there, things aren't working right. In that trapped place, we try to fit in, find help, survive another day.

Luckily for my sanity, deep in my core, I have tried to hold on to the idea that I am here in this body to get a human experience. That I am a spirit. Honestly, when the fog was so thick, and that message about fog came to me that FOG can mean FEAR OF GOD or FEAR OF GOOD, and unfolding my insecure, not worthy belief, it was a big aha! A fog lifter. I think that message has gotten me through. Pretty darn sure of it.

Survival mode. If there is some way that you can truly extract these insights – and use it to help you, not as a knew excuse to give up on life or be a victim or blame ... but school, soul school, then YOU will have something powerful to turn around and teach others.

What I would like to leave this chapter with is if you can find the awareness that you are in survival mode - time and hope are medicines, aside from natural and/or pharmaceutical help, and to be honest about it.

Tell your family/friends what you can and cannot tolerate right now. I apologized so many times I wore out the word - *sorry*. Because I was. I was sorry I could not go to parties. Host a party. Go fly on an airplane. Go to a club. Restaurant. I was sorry that Christmas was so hard to shop, think, wrap, whatever. Holidays became overwhelming.

Believe it or not, the ones that are in your world have the ability to learn something from you. Children are not going to be quiet. Their noise generally is JOY. FUN. They have needs. Spouses have needs. They are not trained caregivers and know nothing about brain injury. But - TV can be turned down. Malls can be avoided. Less instead of more.

Life goes on.   Mine did.   Meals had to be cooked. Animals fed. Bills paid. Parents needed help.   I was fogged. Then it would lift and I was unstoppable, making up for lost time. Then, I was fogged again. And so on. But I did it.

I called bill collectors and said "SORRY" or I overpaid in panic that I would forget to pay.   I was in that fog that was not stuck in a bed paralyzed, therefore I had to function. To look at me, at least in the afternoon, when eye swelling wasn't as present, I looked okay, most the time. I think. Come to think of it, one fog hit, I did not recognize my face in the mirror for several months.

If you are connected to a group, a church, some place where others live to help - want to bring love and helping hands, it has to start with you. Being okay with others helping. I did not want someone to come in and help clean a messy kitchen, because I was embarrassed about THE MESSY KITCHEN. My pride and privacy, in this survival mode, probably slowed my healing process.

My advice, suggestion, encouragement to you - be honest.   It is when you aren't honest that this whole foggy mess gets thicker. Try to stay open to incoming life. Even in tiny doses.   There is a world of unhealthy out there. It is hard to avoid. Sitting behind a diesel engine, any kind of poisonous fumes, new carpet smells, wild parties, alcohol, drugs, pounding and any type of percussion, sugar, heck even dishwasher soaps are often bleach-based. Life changes. A lot. But it can teach too.

Or here is a wacky one, while in survival mode. Fluoride. As crazy as it seems, protecting the enamel on our teeth, findings are showing what fluoride can do to the brain! Go figure.

Survival mode means a lot of things. For me it was doctors, MRIs, medicine trials, emotional roller coasters, disappointment, disillusions, and on and on. That is why I wrote this dude. I wanted to have a way to say, "WHEN THE FOG LIFTS" a deeper life meaning might be waiting for you and maybe those around you.

Depression, anxiety and anger attacks, any mega fears, paranoia and/or hallucinations can be danger. Dangerous to you and your family. So, if you are experiencing any of these, seek help, please. Things happen upstairs in our wondrous brain that can push the wrong buttons. Seratonin levels can drop dramatically with injury. Our "feel good" helper in our brain.

I know a minister who shared that he may never go off of his anti-depression medicine, due to the damage that happened in his brain. He said to survive and thrive by taking a pill, was so much better than dying in the fog. It is a tricky one for each of us to know the right direction. And no one likes to be a guinea pig of meds when fog is already dominating.

I have heard many stories of a low dose medicine can help. I keep my Gabapentin in the cupboard. And still have to take it now and then when multi-firings begin and take over. Will I ever not need them? Hopefully! But, for now, I have em if I need em.

Life is about balance. It isn't all or nothing much of the time. Moderation keeps us out of trouble. Addiction brings us trouble.   I take what I need to take, without apologies, but try not to let medicine own me. Every opportunity I try to replace something with an herb, rebuild with vitamins, amino acids, foods, - I am always open.

My cupboard is full of vitamins, minerals and such.   I will grab White Willow, Ginger, Feverfew, St John's Wort, Tumeric and/or Cat's Claw before I grab Excederin. But there are days, the migraine wins. Herbs not strong enough. Same with mis-firing, multi-tracking zapping brain – I will take 5 HTP, Hops, or my fav, L-Theanine, but if that doesn't do it, a Gabapentin or Lorazapam does. Resets my noodle to rest.

My brain is a creative active computer up there on my shoulders. If I burn it out, that too is injuring it.   I finally understand this.

In survival mode diet really makes a difference. Not waiting all day to eat and messing with blood sugar. Not gorging on sugar. Small nibble meals through the day seem to help. More water, less coffee.

My tiny mama has to take many things to move. She is so full of Osteo with knees completely gone, spine twisted badly, but, that lil gal takes meds so she can function. Riddled with pain, in survival mode, I do not judge her for what she has to live on because without, she would not want to live. She would lay down and die.   Of course I try to share with her anything I can research to help her.   Even in her severe condition, if she can, she will take her little hoe and go outside and pull weeds like nobody's business. Most incredible weed puller I have ever known.   Like a tiny machine. She cannot stand up straight, or walk without support, but she can bend in half like Gumby, and pulverize weeds. At least at the time of writing this. And she is 82 and 3/4s!

So, yes, life is balance. Suicides happen when people are worn out, give up, lose hope or afraid to ask for help. If we replace judgment with love, it is amazing HOW POWERFUL love is.

We might not be able to heal another, but letting them know we care, they will know they are loved. Far too often we get padded expressions. Robotic advice, and so on. But sometimes, folks just do not know what to say. We have to try to thank them for even trying to give a damn! Because they have stuff too!

So, from where I see things, there is hope for deep and meaningful enlightenment yet! Or, at the end, of you reading this big, long-winded book, you will conclude that I am simply full of it!

Ironically sitting and doing this typing stuff, no other way for me to share it, is not natural either. I am not moving spinal fluid. Something my chiropractor said we forget to do. We need to MOVE. Shake it up. Stretch it out. Woohoo!

~

I laughed when I told a friend that I used a "warm" typing font, Comic Sans MS ... perfect for a goof comic like me. He said in a serious tone, "Well, I will let you know what I think." Referring to the chosen font type. My come back surprised me: "I don't care. I like it! It's me!" You don't take 10 years to write a book to worry if one person likes the font!
I think I shocked us both! He meant well. So did I.

This book would have been written MUCH faster had I not had to use spell check so dag gum often, to unscramble some words. Oh my. I just typed speeelchecked and it said, "Whaaaat?" But then, I took a sip of coffee and chuckled as I read my coffee cup that says:

LIFE IS GOOD.

AMEN!

Chapter 43 - A Common Thread

Gosh, once the heart is doing the navigating on a project such as this, to truly want to sprinkle hope into our global need of healing - it can be endless. The more you have experienced in life, the more you can relate to others. Their hurts. Their healing. It bonds us as a common thread.

We are born, we live, we die. That right there is our common thread. What happens on the journey and what we do with it, that's the big part.

Heck, just the fact that most of us breathe on our own, without machines, and even though Dementia and Diabetes are storming our country, we still have choice. We have abilities to research and choose higher roads of health and living. Its all there. All choice.

This little entry is the common thread about brain. The big enchilada that runs the show. I can look at a few key people that I love and honor very much- who have walked this life with me, but also have had a heck of a run with brain. When I think about their lives and what happened to their brains, I think it is worth mentioning.

I want to briefly share on several beautiful people because even with what happened to them, each, in their own way, are pumping out love and light to the world. Each could write their own book!

I won't name them for their privacy, but will bow in honor that they are inspirations and represent MANY, as we all come together to lift fog and LIVE a fuller life.

One incredible woman was camping. The propane on the

heater leaked in the trailer and poisoned her. She was nearly dead. Her husband saved her. Since, daily, her life is different. Life has been a challenge. But her heart is wide and full of love.

One extremely talented, wise teacher, has his own company and also has been speaking on spirituality for decades. He had a huge, grapefruit-size tumor on his frontal lobe. Removing it was deadly. He came through it with a total wake-up call. To live his life connecting to others about oneness. Rather than core focus on ego and money/power.

A long-time friend experienced the perfect storm. Riding on a motorcycle for hours in extreme heat over the mountains, had taken pain medication, got dehydrated and heat stroke. To some degree, one could say she fried her brain. Her husband found her nearly dead in the morning. Rushed to the hospital. Her journey back has been all an equal to any of my injuries. And through it, is an intelligent, beautiful heart in the medical field and has cared for many.

Another long-time dear brother energy, experienced a series of mini strokes. Hospitalized. Unable to speak. Had to walk through the black places of the brain to come back to his fullness. A spiritual author as well, living to touch others lives ... and inspire.

Another friend, while snow shoeing, fell and hit her head.   Then went through a devastating divorce and depression. Treated for mental illness issues.   Not even connecting head injuries.   Still battles with the power of the brain. The darkness. But also holds a special place in my heart. For we have known and seen each other through a lot.

An incredible humanitarian friend, who has been a catalyst and involved with many charitable projects walked through a huge concussion. Living alone, new in town, only a few acquaintances. She definitely understood my journey as we worked on a project together.   Only thing was, her mind was fast, mine was slow.   So we also had some challenges together! She also had to go through the blocks of searching for words, scheduling and committing issues, etc. Not the massive migraines that took me out for days. But other symptoms.   The wondering what was wrong with her.   Waiting to get clear from the fog.

Another dear friend, in a blink of an eye, clobbered in the forehead at a new job, experienced many of the post-concussion stuff, and damaged an eye from the jarring. Still dealing with the eye pain and headaches.   With concussions, often you feel something is actually controlling you, and you are just trying to get by day to day.

Then of course was my dear daddy. He took it all in the course of his life. Toxic poisoning, concussions, stroke... front lobe tumor... dementia.

These loved ones are all in different injury camps, all effecting the brain.   Tumors, concussions, gas poisoning, stroke, dementia. With over 5 million people in the U.S. alone, now diagnosed with Alzheimer's, becoming *mindful of the mind* is the only thing that is going to change those numbers. It is predicted that by 2025 those numbers may be 1/3 higher!

A common thread that would be wise to express here again if you happen NOT to be the injured one, but learning about your son, daughter, spouse, relative, friend, co-worker etc... we are not spared. We can't all have brain injury or this world would collapse.

But those who walk through it are teachers about NOT taking our thoughts and functioning brain for granted. WE do stupid things. We think we are invincible. Drugs, sports with repetitive injuries, poor diets, burn-out. We, in general.   The fact that I lived through my drinking teen days while driving my gal pals around, more shit-faced than them – blows my chips that we lived. That I LIVED.

Each thing we go through can, if we are open to it, connect us. We are not an island. We are the ocean. All interwoven.   Dang, that is so, like, metaphysically deep, I might need to go clean out some horse shit from the barn.

Don't assume you understand another's issues unless you have worn their shoes. But listen. They have something to teach.   They might spare you from this journey just by sharing their wisdom. To them, like me, while in the fog, may feel dumb as a stump!   But they aren't. Help them know that!

I am a big fan of the Willow Tree.
"Whaaaat?" You ask. "Now where the heck is she going?"
Common Thread?

The willow is known for several things. It can be started by simply poking a branch in the ground or water. It will root. It can withstand unbelievable winds. Bending over. If it breaks from high winds or a more likely heavy load of snow, it will grow back. If the branch touches the ground it may even take root. Its bark was the original aspirin for pain. It can be bent in the tiniest of circles when handled while still green, if worked gently, but if forced, can snap and smack ya across the face.   Ah, like life!

Willow can even look dead on the ground and if it gets put in water, can come back to life! The only thing I have known to kill willow is the deepest freeze. I suppose one could say, if they were striving to be like the willow, that when the load gets too heavy or self-care and nurturing cease to exist for too long, one could give up.

A common thread of all of us, is that we can be like the willow. We can learn to bend, withstand high winds of life, come back to life after being cracked, abused, bent too hard. But the critical survival of the willow comes from being flexible. When we fall, we can try to come back to life with a little love and nurturing and be a pain reliever to another, who is enduring their own pain, just by being kind and loving. Or, we can bend and snap, and someone will get slapped in the face.

I do not know how this stuff comes out of my brain. I do not even think about it. I just started typing with A Common Thread in my head. Boom. I believe that we are connected. We can see it once we live from less brain and more heart. Perhaps that is why those with damaged brains become some of the brightest heart-centered beacons for our world. We do not have to get there by damaging our brain. Scientifically, the brain can be dead but the heart will keep beating. But when the heart stops beating, lights out. Life over. Here's to a life of a beating, full-of-love heart!

Regardless of intelligence, wealth status, material stuff – when we come from the heart, fog lifts and a common thread is very obvious bringing more peace and depth to our lives.

You say it, I say it, we say it - see?
We say without thinking: "Twas meant to be."

When something big - we cannot explain,
suddenly happens -walking through pain.

Our faith arrives - taking quiet steps,
in desperate darkness- tears being wept.

We search for the why- through joy, through dread,
connecting our hearts - A Common Thread.
LLL

Chapter 44 - Even If

Through my sharing in the previous words, hopefully I have brought some reality of the pain, sorrow, fear, enlightenment, joy, blessings and wonder what might come next.   It wasn't meant for you to read this and for me to say: YOU will heal and be the exact person you were before. Or your loved one. I was aiming for the reality that YOU/ME - we are growing. Might not feel that way. But I think it is true. It shifts the focus from poor me, to WOW, rich me for learning and growing with this opportunity. If we can feel, in the heart, and connect with others before we die, to me, that makes us rich!
Life is teaching us.

So this is the tricky one, that I live with every day.

Through the years I go to bed at night, often pretty late. Mostly because by 9-11, PM, 12 or even later, I am at my optimum. Whatever works in the brain fluids, spinal fluids, it has been upright long enough to be running through my whole body - instead of morning brain. It feels better. Clearer. Now getting up to take care of critters in the morning, going to bed so late, that is not wise. Hey, I never said I was good at this stuff. I am just writing about it. I suggest you become brilliant at self-care. Then, someday, you will remind me!

I mentioned earlier, that my chiropractor said we don't use our spinal fluid enough. We sit, slouch, type, watch the tube/computer/texting/driving/travel   and our spinal fluid isn't getting moved around through the vertebra as created. Move it. Bend it. Twist it. *Gently*. So if we know that, and we are capable of even a little, then we are deciding NOT to do it. No one else is. If you are bed-ridden, I apologize for that information. Very frustrating.   But, hopefully your caregiver is helping you with this. Sitting you up. Gently turning your back/spine to squish around the spinal fluid that basically gets like jelly. But even more, the latest findings are that it isn't just muscle. It is the entire body. All the connected tissue. Keeping it moving, keeps life in the whole body!

Well here's my thing as I get closer to finishing this book.... I have shared that I went through many hits to my head in 10 years. A hysterectomy that suddenly hollowed out my body of parts that were suppose to make hormones and sanity. Went through mental and physical abuse long-ago that haunted me for years, until I looked at the abuse and realized it was showing me that deep down - I felt worthless. Okay. Got that stuff.

Once I valued me, that worthlessness began to shift. Once I looked at life as school. Experience. Soul growth, if you will, that too shifted and little by little I wanted to stay here on the planet as long as God gives me. I began to find books, speakers, CDs, movies all that fed this worthiness message. Regardless of the information that we have believed about God, melting it all down to its simplest form that God is LOVE. God is GOOD. So whatever package I am suppose to experience, in this life as Laurie, I am grateful.

So then I have to reckon with the fact that with so many head injuries, I am very much vulnerable to re-hits, to neurological stuff down the road because of the neurons and spaghetti up there that has had to rebuild from all my hits.

I choose to be as proactive as I can with stuffing my body with amino acids, good fats, vitamins, herbs, water (sleep) the trickiest one, healthy foods, and give this life the best chance I can. I am a bit like a canary in a cave. Very sensitive. If I drink wine or eat white, sugary stuff, I pay. Inflammation finds me. Fog finds me. So I know what helps and what hinders. It isn't fun when you want to totally slam your face into a hunk of white cake with thick frosting. Or a mountain-size bowl of ice cream - but then, I remember. So in that moment, I choose my health.

Calling this chapter EVEN IF.   Reality, I am writing this book the best I can. I used a font that was easy to read. A bit bigger than many books. I tried to recall lessons that I have learned. Even if, to you, it did not make sense. All with the intention to inspire and bring hope. I can do what I think is right.   So can you. But life still happens. Living with a paranoid "Don't hit again, or don't eat that cookie, or don't plant too much, or, or, or... reality, I will end up however I will end up. I don't want to limit my life. That alone, is a huge FOG! Hopefully if Dementia finds me and I disappear, I will have some cognitive memory at the end of this journey deep inside. Even *if* trapped behind my eyes. Hopefully, if this happens, while I might look blank to others, I can visit some INCREDIBLE memories. Of dancing. Laughing. Crying. Scared. Mourning. Creating. Farming. Music. Knowing I was loved.   I did love. I WAS love.

Whether I am even here on the planet by the time this book reaches you, it's all good. It's very good. I lived. I brought it forth. Not perfect. Not full of big words.   An injured person, lifting fog, sharing about brain injury and life.

So, may I suggest, *even if* ... ask yourself: WHAT AM I LEARNING?   WHAT WAS I THINKING BEFORE I GOT HURT? WHAT CAN I DO WITH THIS EXPERIENCE NOW? HOW CAN I SERVE THIS WORLD WITH MY STORY?

Sometimes, just asking those questions, makes you slip back into your being and own your life. Doctors, medicines, procedures, they can help, but we have way more abilities that we own. This is YOUR life. YOUR journey. YOUR experiences.

If we can let ourselves believe that we are truly Spirits Playing Human, getting human school to have opportunity to know and express LOVE and GOOD - to help our world, we have done our job. How we look at life, no matter how much pain we may endure – down under it all, we will KNOW, that little by little whatever we go through, this KNOWING becomes revealed, when the fog lifts.

When The Fog Lifts... GOD becomes GOOD. Good begins to filter into everything you experience. Even the uglies look different. Even someone dying, we will not just get stuck on mourning and loss, our souls will see that it was their journey. Their time. It's big stuff. I know.

We will see that in order to shift ourselves into this awakening of GOOD, we have to address why the fog rolled in. It is there to slow us down, block our view of what we think life is all about and make us struggle to see. Maybe white-knuckle the steering wheel a bit, dim our headlights, and in that space... unable to see 3 feet in front of you - basically you return to that pinnacle moment as spirit, thinking about coming to earth to become a human. And experience being human.

You cannot see. It takes faith. You have no idea what will jump out in front of you. But you keep moving forward. At some point, you may pull over, rest yourself, and then go again. FOG has many meanings to me. Fear Of God. Fear of Good. Faith Of Good. Faith Of God. Fabulous Outrageous Good. It is your fog. Your journey.

Fog asks us to call on a little extra help. Even some atheists have been know to say: "Help me God" during dire straights. Interesting huh? So, If fog has rolled in for you in your life, to me, it is the way our beings say CHECK IN, something is up. You have become to left-right wing or full of yourself or in rightness mode or forgotten yourself. FOG says slow down, shift is coming. You are bigger than this. Remember? It might be that whisper that you agreed with God, before you got here, that you promise to PAY ATTENTION if fog rolls in. You will remember. The biggest FOG lifter of all? To see OTHERS in the fog, lifting fog too!

Hangin' up my THUMPER nickname now... given it back to the adorable little rabbit in Bambi and sayin, "If you can't say somethin' gooooood, (pause, trying to recall) don't say nothin' at all."

I hope I have said *somethin' good*. Time to go fling horse poop into soil, till it under and GROW something incredible.   That's right. Take it from an organic singing farmer: Good shit produces rich soil. Rich soil produces wonderful foods! I live in THE GARDEN OF MY SOUL.

We are so much more than we think. So much more going on than we see. EVEN IF, we cannot remember. It is worth a try!

Here is to seeing the blessing in our lives.

The next chapter is so very special to me.   While my daughter was going to college, she had to write a paper. A proper documented paper of a factual subject.   The teacher suggested something the student knew well, or perhaps was curious about themselves.

Well, my dear daughter, Callie, chose a subject "mama" sadly exposed her to for many years.   But she is also my testimony, should one ask, that injured brains can achieve good things. They may be limited on energy, focus, commitment and remembering to buy groceries or turn the bathtub water off, but, they can also make an impact in the world, by sharing their stories and bringing HOPE.

What is beautiful about Callie's paper is that it covers the *mechanics* of our brain. Details I opted to let her share in her research. It is the technical part. And beautifully done!

College paper by my daughter - Callie Lewis

May 27, 2017
Hamilton, IDS
Whatcom Community College
A Fragile Mechanism
A look into the brain and the effects of TBI

It helps us solve our math homework, read the instructions in a recipe, stop at a stoplight, and chew our food. The brain is far greater than just an organ. It is a mechanism. The body cannot exist without the brain, thus making it the key to our existence. Being made of many different lobes, which are packed with individual neurons, nerves and receptors, the brain is in charge of every movement of the body. If the head was to be struck, numerous parts of the body could be affected depending on where the brain was hit. People who suffer from traumatic brain injuries (TBIs) can have a long list of side effects that can last for days, weeks, or years. Learning about brain injury helps the injured, and the people surrounding, to have a better understanding of how the brain works and what they can do to cope with TBI.

The Brain. We have used it since the beginning of time to solve problems, organize, and reason with conflict. We use it to read a novel, write an essay, solve mathematical equations, and more. Unlike the other necessary body parts we need in order to go on with our lives, the brain is the most importance because it runs every part of the body. The brain is divided into three important regions: The cerebrum, the cerebellum, and the brain stem, all of which have very important jobs in keeping the body at its best. The cerebrum is the largest part of the brain and acquires left and right sides. It is in charge of many things such as speech, reasoning, hearing, seeing, and learning. The cerebellum appears under the cerebrum and controls movements such as the muscles, balance and posture. Last, the brain stem, divided into three parts: the midbrain, pons, and medulla, regulate many things in the body like temperature, breathing, heartrate, sleeping cycles, digestion, sneezing, and most importantly: connecting the cerebrum and cerebellum.

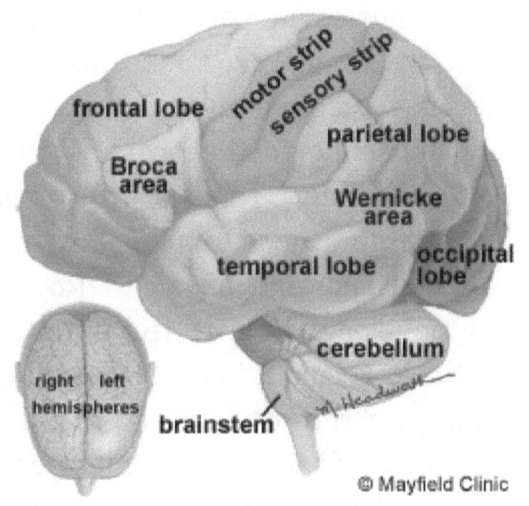

The cerebrum is composed of a right and left side, each consisting of individual lobes that regulate and have control over movements and organs. The left side of the brain controls one's speech, mathematical skills, and writing. The right side of the brain controls creativity, artistry, and musical skills. The brain has four different lobes: the frontal lobe, the parietal lobe, the occipital lobe, and the temporal lobe, each carrying significant roles in the performance of the body. It is important to understand that each lobe of the brain does not function alone. There are very complex relationships between the lobes of the brain and between the right and left hemispheres (M, 2016). The frontal lobe, which sits at the front of the brain, (see figure 1) controls the personality, behavior, and emotions, as well as the ability to speak, write, and problem solve. The parietal lobe has control of understanding language and wording, pain and temperature, as well as vision, hearing and memory. The occipital lobe has control over vision interpretation. Lastly, the temporal lobe, assists in hearing, learning, organizing, and understanding language. The brain, being capable of so many different functions, is an interesting subject when looking at how it works in understanding mathematics, problem solving, and how the brain recognizes symmetric patterns, illusions, and impossible figures.

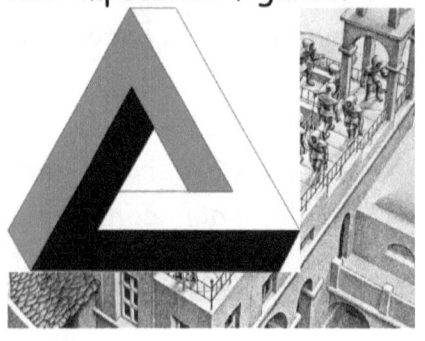

Artists and architects have used geometric structures and mathematics in their work since the beginning of time, and all because such patterns and shapes are appealing to the brain. Artist M.C. Escher, famous for his impossible geometric illustrations, got his ideas from mathematician and physicist Roger Penrose who is famous for the popularization of the artistic triangle (see figure 2). The artistic triangle is an "impossible figure". It is a picture of an object that at first sight looks three-dimensional but cannot be a two-dimensional projection of a real three-dimensional object (Impossible figure, n.d.), such as Escher's drawing of a staircase which visually looks to be going up as well as going down at the same time (see figure 3). How our brains interpret the artistic triangle is the same as how it interprets optical illusions. Our brains are constantly trying to interpret things happening around us, and optical illusions try to trick the brain so that it is unable to comprehend whether something is real, or not.

The brain is capable of so many different things on its own, that the only job as human beings is to keep it healthy, strong, and safe. To protect the brain, we have the skull, and the cerebral fluid keeping the brain cushioned safely within. To take more precaution, it is important to wear head protection such has hardhats when working in a construction zone, or helmets for riding bicycles, a horse, or playing football. Even with such safety precautions, there is no 100% guarantee that the brain will never result in an impact. Helmets break, cars crash, horses spook, and the body may be thrown into a forceful hit, resulting in a Traumatic Brain Injury (TBI).

Whether it happens on a football field or in the safety of your home, a hit to the head can change one's entire life. There are approximately 1.5 million people in the U.S. who suffer from a traumatic brain injury each year. 50,000 people die from TBI each year and 85,000 people suffer long-term disabilities (What is Traumatic Brain Injury?, n.d.). When the skull suffers a hit, the brain is jarred within the skull, being put out of its normal safety cushioning of the cerebral fluid.

Since the brain has different lobes controlling different parts of the body, depending on where the head is hit, can determine what functions may quickly become unbalanced. It does not always take an extreme impact for a brain injury to occur. In simple circumstances, someone could be cleaning their rug, quickly rise up, and clash into a low-hanging lamp. In worse, more traumatic circumstances, someone could get in a car crash and be thrown through the window, resulting in a severe head trauma. To determine the severity of a head trauma, several methods are used. Doctors will often start with a computerized tomography (CT) scan, which takes an overall view of the brain making it easy to see any fractures, or whether there is bleeding or swelling. The next step in looking into the brain is magnetic resonance imaging (MRI) which looks at the layers of the brain to get a more accurate picture of its condition. One of the most reliable way to test the severity of the brain injury on site is through the Glasgow Coma Scale. The Glasgow Coma Scale (GCS) is the most common scoring system used to describe the level of consciousness in a person following a traumatic brain injury. Basically, it is used to help gauge the severity of an acute brain injury (Brainline, n.d.). The Glasgow Coma Scale is used for those who have suffered a severe head trauma such as a car crash or sports accident. The test measures the time it takes to open the eyes (on a scale of 1-4, 4 being spontaneous), the quality of verbal response (1-5, 5 being normal conversation), and the state of motor response (1-6, 6 being normal response). At the end of the procedure, the numbers are tallied and a decision can be made as to how severe the brain injury is.

It is common for TBI to be seen in Pro Football teams such as the NFL. Due to the constant impact on the players, many suffer brain trauma. In a study at the American Academy of Neurology, led by Dr. Frank Conidi, it was reported that more than 40% of retired NFL players show evidence of abnormal brain structures. And on a series of cognitive tests the players took, half showed serious problems with executive functions such as reasoning, problem solving, planning and attention, while 45% had difficulty with learning and memory (Park, A., 2016). There is probably no end to the game of football anytime soon, but it is important to recognize the dangers of playing football, and learning how to cope with its after effects.

Aside from brain injury and ways of measuring it, the number of effects a person can have from a head trauma are endless. Some people that suffer a concussion may not even be aware that they have injured themselves if the effects are not severe. For some, although the initial hit was not very strong, the effects from the hit can be very noticeable, and take a long time to heal. For a concussion categorized as "mild", side effects can include headache, difficulty thinking or remembering, dizziness, or the feeling of being off-balance. Highly patterned surfaces, loud noises, crowded rooms and busyness can also make someone who has suffered a brain injury dizzy and disoriented. For a person who has suffered a severe brain injury the list of side effects is even longer. The most common sign that the head has suffered something more severe is slurred or jumbled speech. Like a stroke patient, someone who has hit their head may not be able to create a clear sentence, or comprehend what you are trying to say to them. If motor skills are effected, and the person is having a hard time walking a straight line, sways back and forth, or feels disoriented on their own feet, it is also a sign that the head trauma they experienced may be more severe then mild.

Memory loss plays hugely into the lives of people who have suffered a head injury. Depending on where the head is hit, and the severity of the injury, a brain injury could affect their immediate, short term, or long-term memory. Immediate memory is used when someone tells a quick fact or opinion, or tells his or her phone number aloud to someone to be written down. The memory lasts long enough for you to understand what is being said or done, but not to retain it for a long period of time. Short-term memory, as said by Dr. Glen Johnson, is the ability to retain something after 30 minutes. For example, someone may tell you to go to the store and get some milk, some eggs, a newspaper, and some dish soap. By the time you get to the store, all that you remember is the milk (Johnson, G., 2010). .Long term memory is used for the things that we remember after days, weeks, or years. Because brain injury affects short-term memory, and long-term memory is based off short-term memory, people who have suffered from a head injury can usually tell someone what happened many years ago, but cannot tell them what happened yesterday. Many who have suffered a head trauma have problems remembering English and mathematical skills. Although much of your basic math is stored throughout the mind, in our long-term memory, it can be affected by getting a concussion. Laurie Lewis, a northwest farmer, and singer-songwriter, has suffered from multiple head injuries in the past, and has had a significant struggle in doing every day math such as addition, subtraction, and multiplication. Laurie said "As a farmer, trying to figure out whether you are making money or wasting it, you are constantly juggling numbers. The most difficult challenge I have had so far, is point-of-sale, at our plant sales. Counting plants and adding by 4's. My mind will go blank. Instead of crying, I have had to learn to simply tell the customer I have math challenges since my concussions and the burden suddenly becomes a blessing, and people are happy to help" (Lewis, L., 2017).

Something peculiar about the human mind is that as common as it is for memory and certain abilities to be lost, there have been several occurrences where someone has benefited from hitting their head, and gained prodigal abilities. Jason Padgett, of Tacoma Washington, was brutally attacked one night in 2002. He suffered from a severe concussion, and PTSD. Although Padgett never had interest in academics, he began being able to see complex intricate geometric shapes and physics concepts with the naked eye.

What Padgett acquired is called "Savant Syndrome", in which people gain prodigal abilities. Most people gain musical or artistic talents, and it is very rare for someone to gain mathematical abilities. After his injury, Padgett was drawing complex geometric shapes, but did not have the formal training to understand the equations they represented. One day, a physicist spotted him making these drawings in a mall, and urged him to pursue mathematical training. Now, Padgett is a sophomore in college and an aspiring number theorist (Lewis, T., 2017). It goes to show that not all brain injuries result in a loss or struggle.

Surviving an accident and getting a head trauma is only the beginning of the journey. Head injuries do not only affect the victim of the trauma, but the people that surround the person such as friends, family, coworkers, the cashier at the grocery store, and anyone else that the person would run into. It becomes what started as just an injury, to a long battle of trying to deal with balance issues, sensitivity to noise, and a number of other things. So, one may ask, how does one with a brain injury cope?

Andy, a former member of the undercover NYPD narcotics force, worked undercover for years in the streets of New York. When he began the program, he was taught how to walk, talk, and forget his own name as to not give anyone the notion that he was an undercover cop. Working undercover is a dangerous job, because if you act out of character even for a split second, it could put you in the position to lose your life. Although Andy worked in dangerous situations every day, the night that would change his life forever had very little to do with his job.

While sitting in his car with his partner awaiting a case, a car flew from around a corner crashing into them. It took several days for Andy to gain the effects of the concussion. Andy was diagnosed with post- concussion syndrome. When things began to be looking up, and Andy had been taking physical therapy, he lost the ability to walk. After re-learning how to walk, his wrist clenched up and was never the same. All was due to neurological imbalances within the brain. Andy says Post-concussion syndrome... a strange thing that does the unthinkable, making you feel like you've lost your mind, your sanity, and, worst of all, the life that you once took for granted. (Braininjurystories, 2016). Andy lost a lot of his memory after the accident and still struggles daily. He says "I will be disabled for the rest of my life, but learning to adapt to the changes, learning to take life a day at a time, has saved me from the grips of depression". Family and friends also played a huge role in Andy's life when he was struggling to keep his sanity. His wife, his kids, his friends and neighbors, made him realize that he had many things to be thankful for and focus on right in front of him.

Unfortunately, there is no go-to treatment for concussion patients. Depending on the severity, the extent of the treatment might be rest, and over the counter pain killers for headaches. For worse circumstances, a doctor might give a patient diuretics while they're in the hospital. Diuretics decrease the amount of fluid in the brain, and increases the urine output. When a head trauma occurs, the brain will often create fluid to in-case the injury, much like when one bruises their elbow and it created a watery sack around the injury. People who have suffered a severe injury are at risk for seizures after the initial accident, and are given seizure medication to prevent any more brain damage. This is especially helpful if blood vessels, compressed by increased pressure in the brain, are unable to deliver the usual amount of nutrients and oxygen to brain cells (Mayoclinic, 2014).

Other treatments for severe head traumas include surgery to remove blood clots, suturing a cracked skull, or creating an opening in the skull to drain cerebral spinal fluid. The treatments available all depend on the severity of the head injury.

The brain is an incredible organ, made up of many sections all having control over very important parts of the body. Without the brain, we would simply not be. How the brain reacts to mathematical equations and figures is still being explored, as there is always something new for one to learn. How artists have used impossible figures to try to "trick" the brain is a remarkable concept on its own. Although doctors know endless things about the brain, there will always be new things to discover. Being the most important part of the body, one has to try to keep it safe and secure; otherwise, one may result in a traumatic brain injury.

Although we cannot always protect the brain at every moment, it is important to have knowledge of TBI if it ever becomes a problem in one's life. Learning about the effects of brain injury could not only help the person who has gotten injured, but will also help the people surrounding that person to give a better idea of what is happening, and how they can help. Living with a brain injury is not easy, but having a better understanding will make it easier to get through.

References

Braininjurystories. (2016, November 1). Andy's Story. Retrieved May 27, 2017, from https://braininjurystories.org/

Brainline. (n.d.). What is the Glasgow Coma Scale? Retrieved May 27, 2017, from http://www.brainline.org/content/2010/10/what-is-the-glasgow-coma-scale.html

Impossible figure. (n.d.). Retrieved May 27, 2017, from http://www.dictionary.com/browse/impossible-figure

Johnson, G. (2010). Memory. Retrieved May 27, 2017, from http://www.tbiguide.com/memory.

A poem for my Callieflower

You were there in mama's fog
your love is what got me through -
Sayin, "Mama, it will be okay."
I would not be here, without you.

You helped me hold on, when I was weak
you gave me sunshine through the clouds -
We laughed and danced - to Josh Turner
and sang his songs so loud!

Getting a daughter to love - like you
Bouquets, rainbows and songbirds!
Callieflower, I love you so much,
God blessed me, beyond ANY words!

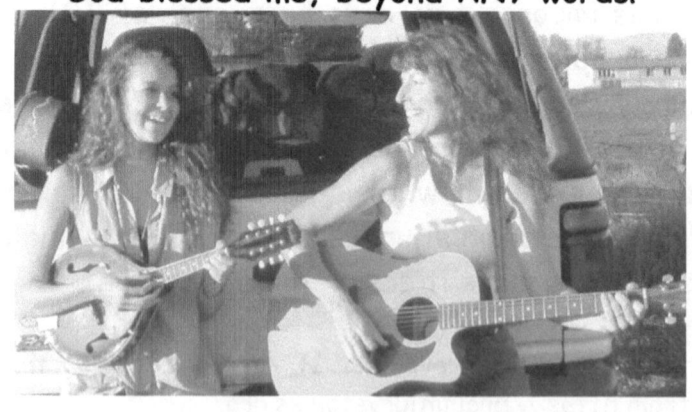

I love you.
Mama, Mom, Mum, Mummy and Madre`

Chapter 45 - The END. The BEGINNING.

Thought I was all done. Thought I had written everything I could remember, and what I have learned from spending large amounts of time in the fog. Shining a love light of hope on any brain fog - be it: injury, mentally or physically, aging, dementia and disease, fog of chemo, hormone and thyroid off-balance, loss, grief, any trauma, menopause... and the list goes on.

Basically, if you have gotten through life without knowing fog, you are a rare brain. I would say that I envy you, but it seems to be the law of balance - that helps us learn one lesson from another. The opposites. Contrast. So no fog, will you really know clarity... and appreciate it? Maybe. This much I know, as I watch myself get healthier, I cherish every moment. I never take clarity for granted!

What I did not realize about this book was something that could not have been written until I experienced New Year's eve weekend, 2017. God has the coolest ways of working with my brain, foggy or clear when I ask for help. I had asked to finish *When The Fog Lifts*, so I could move on. To END it, so I could have a new BEGINNING.

We get through foggy stuff and are grateful, *hopefully*, and then a bit of amnesia can set in. Kinda forgetting the whole dark detail back then and the cry for help. The ego wants to flip back and take control to that place we were before - we cried out. When you are really out there, lost in fog, it is the time, if you are spiritual at all, or inching that way, to a deeper meaning of life – where God comes into focus. The secret is – holding on to your gratitude and remembering your *cry out*. Your *surrender*. Your *faith* or newly found *faith*. Your *purpose*. Seeing *blessings* instead of *bitchings*.

Sometimes, people have a very strong faith and then something tragic happens and they lose it. Their mother suffers a painful, long death. Dementia takes their father's brain but not his body. Suicide takes a sibling or friend. Where is God then? Or you smack your head and everything you knew - changes. Your cool marriage collapses and you have to start all over again.   Somehow... when life seems darkest, a flicker of hope tells you to hang on. There is something more.

In the simplest form, I have always seen God as *love*. My mom taught - from that place. Oh, sometimes she would pull the guilt card, *GOD IS WATCHING YOU, Laurie!* Aka punishment, which was freaky and hard to understand. Especially stretching my teen wings to experience smoochin' at a movie or drunk-as-a-skunk, wondering how I got home. Maybe God *was* watchin'... cuz someone drove us home! That is what my mom was taught.

The day, however, that I heard mom *guilt out* my little daughter this way, (my greatest gift from God) I put my foot down and said, "No more. No guilt teachings about LOVE and GOD. That is YOUR version of God, mom, not mine." Ya know what? It worked. Mom stopped! Who'da thunk!

Aging, surviving, experiencing some healing from deep pain and fog, I found myself as a soul surrendering to say: I cannot run this ship alone. It is dark in here. PLEASE TAKE THE WHEEL. Let's try it your way. Wait? You need more from me? You need me to let go of my crapola, vices and victim mentality? Whaaaaat?! Yah but...

Demanding to God is funny. It is really *you* surrendering control, and for some folk, that is not easy or even cool. There is a ping pong ball energy, bouncing back and forth that goes something like: *HELP ME GOD, PLEASE. I believe. Halleluiah! But then, alright, I am healed! Okay back to me now.* Oh shoot, something else just happened and its once again: *GOD, I need you again...* and so on. Ping... pong... ping... pong.

I have been reading and listening to the motivational spiritual teacher/author, Marianne Williamson for a long time. You can go to her website and sit in on her live-stream services every Tuesday. Her teachings are based on the non-religious writings called: *A Course In Miracles.* I swear, every time I would be in the ping pong game, and tuned in to her teachings... there she was - nailing the very issues and questions that I had! Wow! But with LOVE, not guilt! Although she does end her talks with a powerful Matriarch wisdom by telling us we need to rebuild this world by returning to love.

Marianne offered a beautiful 3-day gathering to reboot our lives going in to 2018. I did not have the funds or a farm sitter to fly to L.A., stay in the motel and afford the seminar. I was alone during the holidays except tending to my folks, so I asked if I could apply for a scholarship.

To my absolute delight, I received an email saying YES, I would be able to attend all 3 days, from the comfort of my farm, for free. Folks, I cannot tell you how incredibly inspiring this woman's heart and passion are - for rebuilding our world through love. To let go and heal our pasts, honor what we are now, and move into becoming miracles. Essentially the earth angels to off-set the balance of hate, greed and power - that dominates this world. Face our fog and lift it!

Marianne took us through the first day, of looking at guilt, sorrows, grudges "baggage". Looking at our own actions. Truly saying LOOK. Go there. But then, she said, if you could believe that God or love – (whatever fits your comfort language) – will take it away, release it, if we are willing to

LET GO. To release. To forgive yourself. To ask for forgiveness. To see yourself as you truly are. A perfect spirit. And, to glean from those so-called mistake/experiences.

Boy did this hit home. I thought about how if someone complimented me, I never knew how to respond. I did not want to seem arrogant, ever! Nor, did I ever truly feel like I wrote or produced songs that were as good as most.

It seemed I attracted *some* people in my life that would affirm my deep belief that I was not good enough. *Truth is, I was just bouncing my own low self esteem off of them - so I could blame someone.* Takes some *deep* searching to come up with that and *own it*. Especially with an altered brain!

My middle brother was pretty pissed that I was born. Took mama's love from him. I was humpty dumpty fatty, big-headed baby girl, that grinned. A lot. Mom said I was a happy baby. But slowly - that changed.

My dad drank til I was about 24, when he quit cold turkey. He could be pretty funny, til he got into a swearing fit or embarrassed us at parties and such. But the harder part was having this brother that despised me. I was shy just like him. I would turn beet red whenever mom insisted that I sing a song for family, because she was so proud. It only seemed to make him hate me more.

When someone you admire, as I did to my bigger brother, I thought his words were true. Calling me show off, or *idiot* for years, I thought I *was* an idiot. Sadly, words are poisonous. Most of us don't have the tools to understand another person's fears and insecurities that come out on you, when we are young. Or even grown up, for that matter!

The fog I knew back then - was that for some reason, from my perspective, my bro hated me. When I finally asked my mom why, she answered, "Because you were born." Now, I don't know about you, but without enough good explanations to help a kid understand, that one sucks! Aka: fog to lift, years down the road!

Marianne's words burned through me, about letting go. Looking at my actions. Looking at false words that we wear. And then: Letting go. Letting go. Letting go. Letting go!

To rise up and be a bright, beaming light for the world.

That light, and calling my worthiness forth, kept showing up for me to grow.   I stumbled into modeling and recording music. Once this started, I felt that I could not relate to family – as if they saw me differently. I always had a ceiling on how far I would let myself go in success. Something always haunted me. In fact, when I was living in a stinky, cold attic in Seattle with rats, and very hungry, I felt like I deserved it, because I was trying to survive as a model. HA! Nobody knew the truth.

I forgive my brother for that stupid stuff. I get it now.   At some point, when you are called to use your talents and gifts, with an "I must do this" pull, you have to step beyond that past. Somehow stop worrying what others think. The END can become the BEGINNING - when you let go.

Ironically, there was almost a relief when my brain got scrambled. *Almost.* A reckoning that said, "There God, now I cannot do the things you gave me to do. See, I am injured. Can't even speak without a stutter. Can't remember how to play guitar or remember words to songs. Bummer God. No more pressure. Whew." Call Reba, she is already in the spot light! She can do big things! Ha! Right! No free lunch for me!

So back to the part of Marianne. She took us through some big stuff. Asking us to go back. Forgive yourself, forgive others. Then, ask to be healed. She referred to the inside power we all have. Some call the holy spirit, or a deeper knowing, gut feeling, insight or whisper.

She spoke of being miracle workers by getting out of the way, (our ego) and let God/love - use us as instruments of peace. That takes a mega dose of courage and release to say: *Okay, I think I get the being small part.*

When you are healing from brain injury, and you feel trapped in a time capsule, suspended, not sure if the fog will lift, spirituality - is another medicine on a cellular level. Going within. Shutting off the world outside. Try some meditating to a quiet place. In that space, simply asking: HEAL ME PLEASE. SHOW ME what you want me to do with my life. If you aren't a praying or meditating type, heck, talk to the air! If there is a loving universe/God, and you are sincere, wonderful things begin to happen! Amazing stories.

We all walk our own path, learning and growing. It is what we do with the growing - that makes all the difference. I admit, during heavy fog, post-concussions, there is no way I could have tracked an online talk. I would have become agitated, dizzy and nauseated. The brain would not have understood, nor could I have held attention or information. But, but, but, THIS New Year's weekend, I was gifted this seminar. I was smiling, crying and giving thanks and that I could DO IT!

I thought I had written enough for this book. But then, Marianne showed me that I had not. I still carried around a truck load of stuff. Old pain. Old grief. Old grudges. And in reality, during a meditation that she held, I saw my depths of pain and fear. Holy moly! Plus, what I could not foresee, was how apparently I was then suppose to go through the rapid decline and passing of my dad, who battled Dementia. To include in the book.

During Marianne's beautiful meditation, suddenly I heard the voices, over 10 years, of folks asking about my head hits. Asking me if I had a death wish, self torture, knocking sense into myself... etc. (because I kept hitting.) I watched of how mad that made me. Then I heard: *accidents are NO accidents and, if you get it, the fog lifts.* WOW! It was like a *Field Of Dreams* - movie moment. "Free *HER* Pain."

I knew I had to share this part, about LETTING GO OF IT ALL. Thanking my injuries. Thanking those who I felt hurt me. Thanking God for my life. Thanking all those who care about me. Thanking those I did and did not feel judged by. I think you get it. There was a whole lotta *thankin'* a goin' on! (envision a bit of curled-lip, Elvis attitude, there!)

It was an intense weekend. Doing the work with Marianne. Firing up for the new year. As a servant of light. Of love. But what happened at 12:05 A.M. Jan. 1st, was transforming.

No matter how fired up you can get with stuff like this, *doubt* and *fear* love to show up and nibble on your ass, when you decide bust through the fog and become your authentic self. To go as far as calling yourself a MIRACLE WORKER, as Marianne said. WHOA. Letting God or LOVE, whatever is comfortable to read here, to use us to work together, to build a better world. Another WHOA.

The gathering ended with meditation and fantastic music. Then, I went outside. I had yet another experience.

I wrote something on Facebook later that day to share, in which, I decided to copy and paste here:

Happy New Year! I just finished a phenomenal online seminar weekend, with motivational speaker/author, Marianne Williamson. After dancing at midnight in the living room with my Buster Brown dawgy - in my jammies, bathrobe, scarf, pink hat, Levi coat and boots... Buster and I went outside at 12:05 A.M. Glistening white frost and a big, beautiful moon beamed down and lit the way for us to crunch on frozen grass to the end of the property. 15 degrees. Everything twinkled. Still.

My little farm stand had its own halo. The tilled soil lay quiet and frozen. The Little Redneck Chapel welcomed the two of us. The mossy-sided little building, the cross on the door, the moonlight peeking through the old window.

I lit 4 candles, for: peace hope, healing and joy. My Buster dawg laid by my feet. Soft booms of fireworks echoed off the mountain. We sat there a long time. Thought about life. Thought about change. Thought about the shackles that hold souls back from being happy . Excuses. Sorrow. Ailments. Fear. Worrying what others think. And I said, "NO MORE. Lift Fog Lift." I sat quietly and this is what came to me:

To shine your light for the world ... to inspire - is not arrogant. To believe we each have an assignment to wake-up, to do our part to reset the world, starting in our own being - is being responsible members of the big family. It's not about me. It's not about you. It's about US. It is time to stop apologizing for gifts, talents.

If we let go of our old story, take what we have learned and use it, change has to happen. It is cause and effect. Love grows love. Hate grows hate. Hate isn't workin'! I choose to lift my fog and be love in action.

While you may never read this, Thank you so much, Marianne, for your powerful, authentic work you do endlessly - to lead us back to ourselves. To help us remember and build a NEW world. I hope you become our 2020 President and take us back to our ethics and values! Love, Laurie

When we are willing to let go and END the story of the past, fog lifts, and new BEGINNINGS emerge.

Chapter 46 - BLACK HOLE

Like life, this book unfolds in a weird order. I did not intentionally take you to fog-lifting moments, then drop you back into heavy-load stuff on purpose. But, life is like that. Highs, lows and sideways! Catching us off guard. Now this part, this, is hard to write. But I think it is a critical part of the fog.

The black hole. I have mentioned it several times. AKA: Depression. The darkness. It can hit a head that has never been injured. It can hit even harder when it has. Suddenly, TEARS. Suddenly, I DON'T WANT TO LIVE ANYMORE. Suddenly, I CANNOT DO THIS CORRECTLY. Suddenly, the pull of ... the BLACK HOLE.

How does this happen when you were steady and fine the day or hour before? I have tried to write this book as if we are in the living room, sharing our deepest heart stories. Taking off the masks. Being *really* real. And so it is on this trip down the Black Hole of depression.

Day to day, with or without injury, we are trying to hold it together. Whatever life is throws at us. But darkness might be climbing the pant legs - just waiting. When we aren't living life present and aware... the black hole is easier to fall into. Just waiting for the distracted one. All seems to be going well, then boom! UGH! Something small might be all it takes.

Anyone who knows depression and darkness knows the black hole. With brain injury it may pull harder and faster. One step and down you go, losing your balance. Solid ground begins to give way... and you drop.

Mentally you may feel like your fingers are making claw marks on the sides as you sink. The pull on your feet taking you down is strong, your grip is weak. What will turn this nightmare around? You may have been here before. This time, will the black hole win? Where are you God? HELP!

Chemically things may be popping upstairs like a poison. The darkness is so lonely. Maybe you are not strong enough to tell someone or bother them. Suddenly, your clinging fingers ... let go. Down, down the dark, lonely hole you fall. Your body feels so heavy. Tears. Where did the light go?

On the sides of the walls - passing you by and above you - are images. Your family. Your friends. Your bills. Your home. Your pets. Your beliefs. Your knowledge. Your interests. Your grief. Your dreams. Your grudges. Then, suddenly you stop falling. Suspended. Okay, well, frankly... I didn't want to freak you out - so I hit the pause button. So take a deep breath. I am going to type these words for a few minutes:

Brain injury - always sounds so permanent. If I said back or foot *injury*, we automatically get the message that it will heal. But brain, is our computer. We cannot take out the hard drive and put it in another head and hit the power button. Same brain, is what tells our back or foot that we have pain. That is why our country is full of Opioid addicts. Pain medicines tell the brain: *We aint no got pain!* Then, for depression, we have anti-depressants that tell the brain: *We aint got no pain.* Then, if we cannot sleep and have insomnia we have medicines that tell the brain: *We aint no got pain!* Amazing isn't it? How can we possibly know what is real?

Each person handles pain differently. But if we only medicate and not ever deal with or question our pain, Even if we have to medicate, pain is trying to tell us something.

This writing is called the BLACK HOLE because some of

314

you will read it, and know exactly what I am talking about. Others who have never felt depression, this is also for you. This is to help in your understanding of huge layer of FOG.

So, now I am going to take the pause button off – where I left us suspended, with images going by, falling down that dag gum black hole. *Oh God here it comes:*

The overwhelming darkness. As the walls of your life in the black hole pass you by... you brace yourself for the crippling end. Preparing to hit bottom. Hoping it goes fast. But with depression - it isn't fast. It tortures. Makes you recluse. Blame yourself. Blame others. You wait. You hope the flicker of faith that you had when life was going good - will be the beams of light that will come streaming down the black hole. A hand of love will suddenly reach and lift you back up.

But, how can it? Nobody knows you that you have fallen into this black hole. You did not tell anyone. Perhaps you were wearing the *Happy mask* or the, *I-am-fine mask.* No one knows you are at the bottom. No one sees the thoughts of wanting to die. Wanting to go blank. To release the pain.

Maybe you hear old recordings in your darkness "Just give it to God. You are what you think. Call on God. You are not alone." Then you hear the *horror* voices of those from the past: "Who do you think you are? You're such a phoney. You just want attention." The haunting stories flood your brain.

So you close your eyes and cry out, "GOD HELP ME, PLEASE! PLEASE! Please lift me out of this black hole fog!"

Maybe you reach out while falling, scratching the sides trying to slow down. Once again, crying out: "I feel so alone. God, are you really there? Are you even listening, big almighty God? I am falling fast here!" As you give up... perhaps you hear the whispers: Dear child:

"YOU CAN DO THIS. YOU CAN TURN THIS AROUND. YOU

CAN BE SUCCESSFUL. YOU CAN INSPIRE. YOU AREN'T TOO OLD. YOU CAN HELP OTHERS. YOU CAN HEAL."

The falling body begins to slow down, listening to the whisper. The heavy pull let's up. Are the rays of light about to appear? But then, the black hole begins to pull again screaming: "YOU ARE A LIAR! YOU CANNOT DO ANY OF THAT! YOUR BRAIN DOESN'T WORK RIGHT. IT IS TRICKING YOU. IT IS ALL GOING TO BACKFIRE. YOU WILL MAKE MISTAKES. YOU ARE NOT WORTHY!"

Do you know this story as your read it?
Depression can be very powerful!

Remember, I am writing this and I have been down that hole. Several times. But something pulled me back up - to be here.

I said at the beginning, that writing this chapter was hard to share. And at any moment all I have to do is highlight and delete this whole thing. Why would I want you to read all of that? Simply opt not to include this. After all, this book is about lifting fog, not falling down a damn black hole. Right? But if I don't share, then I have left out a critical voice of this brain injury experience stuff. DOUBT. FEAR. Finally... SURRENDER. Surrender is where the rays of light enter.

Suicide from Brain Injury is on the rise. If you watched the movie *Concussion*, it showed several football players taking their life because their fog never lifted. It won. They felt crazy. Their brains were altered yet they were expected to get back in the game. Feed their families. Pay bills. Fulfill contracts. But in the end, the fog won.

The dark night of the soul. The black hole. The stories that say: when you hit the deepest bottom, there is no place to go - but up. For some, to truly know the "light" - the contrast from knowing darkness - changes their lives forever.

Well, the only reason you are reading this book, providing you have stuck with me on my wacky writing style, is because the darkness has not won. I know, without a shadow of a doubt in my soul, that every word is true.

If you have fallen into a black hole, and if no one knows you suffer from depression, they may not see you fall. If I can leave one thing here, and I know it takes energy and courage to do so ... please, tell someone. Do not be ashamed. Neurologically, following brain injury, depression is a huge symptom. Seek help. I know it is lonely. I know.

What darkness and fog show me is that even when I think I have got it together, how the scale can tip and I can get lost. Either giving too much time to others, or ego kicks in to try to do too much on my own. Slowly I am learning to stop, reflect and give thanks. I still have a hard time asking for help, but trying. Also, to ask myself: How present am I? Am I way out in front of myself or dwelling on the past? And if I am not paying attention, that is when I have hit my head. And as for black holes... watch where I step! Around here on the farm, it's dog or horse shit, but it can also be black holes!

As mentioned about the dark night of the soul, many great writers say their life-changing wake-up call came at the bottom of the black hole. They will often attach that it was "meant to be" as if their spirit sent them a fax, text, email or call - saying, "Hey you, WAKE UP! You are fogged-in because you are asleep. You have decided to believe what others say, vote what others vote, judge what others judge. You have fallen into the sleep-walking, robotic line." But you had left God/Universe/Spirit a memo on your file, that said, "PLEASE, I don't want to sleep through this life. I want to be fully awake, connected to source/spirit while getting this human experience. Send me a light. Send me a hand. Pull me out of this black hole of self- sabotage, abuse, ego-driven, power-gain, unhealthy body or depressed suicide thoughts. Please help me up, so I can shine my light."

Many cry out: HELP ME GOD - while in the black hole. Why only then? Perhaps because our ego then likes to take control and say, "There, I got through that. All better. Back to old patterns and forget that we survived." It doesn't take long to forget. So, when the fog lifts, HOW do we hold on to our wake up call? Our healing? The blessings?

Sometimes all we need to save us, is to see at the top of the black hole - a bit of light. That light seems to come from surrender and gratitude. If you can think of just ONE thing you are grateful for. Start there. A child. A parent. A brother or sister. A friend. A partner. A pet. A neighbor Chocolate! Coffee! Sex! Music! ANYTHING! Just start with something. I write this because I know this. So as you find even a little gratitude, the falling can slow to a stop.

In the darkest hour, what I feel has kept me here - is thinking of the goodness in my life. My daughter. (My beautiful gift from God.) A child I never imagined I could have. My hilarious, loyal, seriously velcro'd to mama, dog! Dirt. Wonderful dirt. Growing food and flowers. Music.

When all hell breaks loose, I try to quiet my soul enough to stop fighting for control or answers. It is easy to not want to be present in the black hole of depression. But what if, the black hole, is actually like a mirror. It is telling us that depression has arrived, a big fog... *once again* to remind you/me - that we are off balance. Too left or too right. Full of opinion, anger, blame, resentment... Too busy.

What if we can release that heavy load on the shoulders pulling us down. What if we can help lift fog and depression, not by running from it, but by facing it. By recognizing that it is trying to help. To show that: *TOO MUCH - IS TOO MUCH.* Could depression be another wake-up call, saying instead of medicate – look, listen and release?

As I release and feel myself truly let go... of the

darkness, by quieting myself through mediation, prayer, or nature, it is in this gift to myself, little streams of light start to appear at the top of that black hole. The loving hand that may arrive to pull me out - could be through a friendly knock at the door. A call. A smile from a stranger. Kindness where you least expect it. A glimmer of HOPE. A loving nudge from a pet. Or, deciding to GIVE and help another... and in that place, we begin to help ourselves.

As Marianne Williamson and all the great motivational speakers teach: God needs us to fix this world. Using us as instruments of peace, love and hope. When we turn our lives around and use them for service, we shift. Life changes and FEAR OF GOOD goes away, replaced with: FULL OF GOOD.

When we once again become aware of our fog or black hole of depression ... and can absorb yet another experience and see life as a gift – that is when the fog lifts.   So here is to bright, orange sticky notes left along our trail of life, that we posted ahead of being born - warning us: **CAUTION black hole ahead - please use detour and find something to be grateful for!**

This was hard.   It is hard to go deep and then be able to get back out.   I pray that I made some sense here, and brought a little light into the dark. I will admit, for a split second of writing all of that, the wave of: GOING INTO HIDING - once this book is out, came through my fog-lifting noggin'. It took courage to write.   Now to stand tall and say: I AM HERE, grateful for this LIFE... to LIVE, LOVE, LAUGH, LEARN and ... GIVE!

Whew. This is one of those chapters that would be really good to take a break from, move your spinal fluids. Hydrate up. Wiggle and giggle. YUP YUP YUP!

Keep me present. Keep me safe.
If I must, I will tell another
that I am falling, into a black hole
I need a sister or brother.

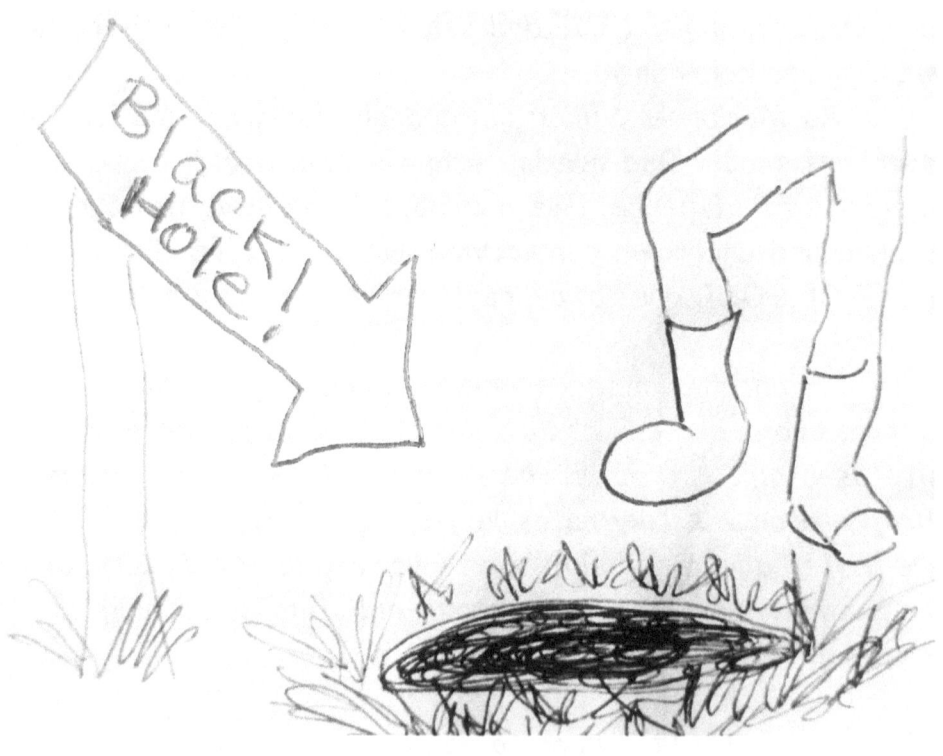

Someone who cares, who will not judge
to reach down and take my hand -
to be the light - in my darkness hour
through love, they'll understand.
LLL

Chapter 47 - Chatty Patty and Busy Lizzy

After each chapter that I have written, I've been pretty dang sure that *that* was plenty. Maybe even too much. So coming up with a goofball chapter like Chatty Patty and Busy (bizzy) Lizzy is beyond me of what my fingers want to tell you. So here we go:

A time-lapse camera sure would be interesting to show just how many times over 10 years that I said, "FORGET IT! I can't think, much less write a book. Let alone figure out about marketing or promotion on a book about brain injury!" After writing some of this, I would close the computer and say, "Maybe, if meant to be, it will come to me." Sometimes, life is too busy to even try to think and focus on such a project. AHA I think I know where this chapter is going!

REAL LIFE, RIGHT HERE... showed me yet another example, challenge, frustration (and exhaustion) for those healing or dealing with brain injury. In reality, any time you are in mega stress or grief mode, brain injury aside, too much, can simply be *too much*. Where, "less is better" is good medicine for sanity and survival! Later, I will talk about toxins. Another fog.

Have you ever found, yourself trying to talk with someone and it goes poorly? It can be exhausting if you get those folks that are good at: rushing you, finishing your sentences, declaring that they know exactly what you mean, or stealing your sentence and then running in their own direction. Leaving you stymied as to what de hell you were about to say!

Oh, and what about that one person who talks *endlessly* who doesn't even check in if you are listening, ever!? Even worse if that person happens to have a tone that is a bit like fingernails on a chalkboard. Oh man. They interrupt. They sound like nonsense. They fill the room with chatter. Ah, Chatty Patty. Note: to any Patty that reads this, no offense. It just rhymed!

Many caregivers mention that this particular person may be the elderly that they are caring for. Non-stop. Talk, talk, talk. Perhaps, silence is a scary thing to them. Its like death whispering, "Yo, I am comin' for ya if you are quiet!" Or perhaps they are very lonely so they just burst with a listening ear, and you are the recipient. This alone for unpaid, 24/7 caregivers of family, can about fry the noodle. I know. I got one. At least at the time of this writing. My lil half-pint, still firing on most cylinders, 82-year-old mama. She loves to tell me that I work too hard outside on the farm. (Bahahaha) aka where the silence is!

Then, either someone else, or maybe that same person might also be a Busy Lizzy. Fidgety. Hyper. Cannot sit down or sit still. So much to do. So little time. Here you are desperately needing YOUR ZEN, quiet and calm. Like I do in the mornings. But instead - have to carry on a conversation that you don't honestly care about, don't want to talk about or give a rip what is on the news... oy yoy!

Add Chatty Patty and Busy Lizzy together, whoa. Anger, anxiety, exhaustion, they can easily show up if this is a steady diet that you feel trapped in. So, hey, spinning the bottle a bit here... IF YOU are the brain injured and it pushed or thumped the chatty or busy in YOU... this might be YOU. See how this wacky school of life works? But if you are the caregiver of the brain injured and happen to be that Busy Lizzy, Chatty Patty, take note. Less is more. Hmm just occurred to me, duh, you might be a guy reading this and saying, "Hey what about Smarty Marty and Bitchy Mitchie!"

You may find that you want to straight out say, "I CAN'T TALK ANYMORE ABOUT THIS or TO YOU." Honestly – this is true. Care-giving my mom, I walk this fine line frequently. So what do ya do?

Well, you can feel guilty. You can get mad. You can ignore. You can try to tell the truth, like: "Hey, not feeling to good and gonna rest." In reality, that person may or may not be able to get it and change. But ya know what? It is worth trying. Start as lovingly as possible, maybe even preface, "I am going to say this as lovingly as possible" and then try your best to say that you need more quiet time. Or not use to talking so much and it is exhausting. The worst thing is to lose it and beller out: SHUT THE F - UP! There is no win/win in that explosion. NO, I have not done that. Ooooh tempting.

In the realm of trying to learn from and lift *fog* ... if you try from honesty, that the healing brain may not be able to handle the noise or busy – at least they may try to be supportive. Or, they will feel sorry for themselves and pout. No guarantee here, but you tried. Good on ya!

This felt worth putting in the book. Cuz if you don't do or say something to a Chatty Patty, Busy Lizzy, or the male version, that unsettled soul energy will come out somewhere through you. Maybe not to them, but someone. Driving. Ordering or shopping. On the phone. At the dog or child. Or, it will cause more fog and like me, you'll hit your head again. Somewhere, someone will get it.

This stuff takes courage, patience and truth. At the end of the day, if your busy chatty person can't hear or they too have brain injury too, um, well? Take a walk. Count to 10. Breathe deeply. Get some help and go see a movie!

Chatty Patty and busy Lizzy
were hanging out one day -
finally Lizzy declared to Patty,
"I need you to go away."

"You exhaust me with all your words,
I need silence and have to do work!"
Chatty Patty got very upset -
and said, "FINE you unsettled jerk!"

The two best friends parted ways
til one day they both hit their heads-
then a funny thing done-did occur
the two met in a store, and met Fred.

Fred was non-stop chatting to the ladies
as he buzzed around busily - as a clerk,
Chatty Patty and Busy Lizzy
tried to escape this Fred - at work.

Escaping Fred, coming out of the store
the two met eye to eye.
Both had headaches and needed to get home
then both began to cry.

Busy Lizzy said to Chatty Patty
"I'm so sorry what I said to you."
Chatty Patty looked at her friend
and with JUST two words, said "ME TOO"
LLL

Chapter 48 - On The Road Again

For some of us, recovery means getting behind a car of life and turning on the key. Remembering how to put it in drive or 1st gear, if a manual, and accelerating forward. Not popping the clutch and killing the engine. Not actually getting it in reverse and running into or over something or someone!

Whoa baby! Where are these fingers going in this writing? I can hear Willy Nelson's song playing in my mind as we set out on this writing journey. "On the road again"...

So, On The Road Again. This can go any direction you choose to take it... but it is all about re-entry into life. To love again. To trust yourself or another again. To be honest. To literally drive. Go back to work. Get a new job. Move. Give up drinking/drugs, toxic thinking. WHATEVER road you find this writing.

The other day, this was me. A bit foggy from no sleep and another thump. My mom and I had conflict regarding finances and me caring for her 24/7 without help or pay. Primarily because I suddenly have no life or income of my own. No income because of being here to help her and cleaning up her home where she and dad lived for 63 years. No help on major decisions about the future. OKAY... got that out of my bitchin' basket. I needed space between my ears and my farm/mom/responsibility. So I took a drive.

During this past winter, cold and nasty, I had 2 cars break down at night with my mom in them. Talk about panic. Then, my car busted a Serpentine belt that runs the whole dag gum car... in pouring rain, pitch dark, smoke coming out, no headlights or power steering, coming home from town.   So trusting my vehicles and my stress levels have been severely tested.   As I headed south merging on the I-5 freeway, cars flying by, I became aware of my ... needed CALM.   My head. My aloud prayer that said, "Please protect me, God. I need this drive and I am *not* completely with it."

I left being present (as you should be driving) and went backward into the past. Not very far. The day before, where I found myself checking the oil on all the cars. The radiator for anti-freeze. The brake fluid. Charging batteries. The transmission fluids. (Although you have to check that when the engine is hot and in park to get an accurate reading.) Oops, forgot tire pressure. Such a feminine, girlie life I live. Lol!

I reflected on a story my dear, DEAR construction and mechanic co-heart friend and fatherly- figure, the one and only, Mr. Marvin - told me. (Marv, was one of dad's besties for the past 10 years or so - of his life.) We both lost our great guy. Soon after dad's passing, we started remodeling mom's house and working on ALL the vehicles and farm stuff, left to my care.

We laughed and healed together as we tried to find tools in dad's garage and barns, worked to sell dad's old tractor and so on. I even made funny videos of our work together. He was so cool when I would just break down and cry.

Marv, perhaps the most sought after intuitive mechanic in the area, for more that 50 years of his life. Still today, over 80, anyone needing a lawn mower or weed eater fixed, finds Mr. Marv. We have needed each other during this window, for he too, had lost his beloved wife just 2 years prior. Now, here he has been, handing down some pearls of auto and construction wisdom and laughter - to me.

His story, as I remembered it, was of a young lady that pulled into his driveway one day en-route to go skiing up at Mt. Baker. She was all stressed and her car was screaming. Marv popped the hood, asked if she had checked the oil. She came back with, "No. Daddy bought me this car 2 years ago, and I have never checked it. Can you fix it and so I can go skiing now?" Marv came back with, "No, your engine is blown up. It needed oil!"

Getting back on the road of life, checking out the mechanics of a vehicle - is a pain in the butt. Preparing for emergencies is also a pain in the butt. Especially if you have just become able to barely bend over and tie your shoes!

This preparedness message ran through my brain loudly, while taking this little jaunt. It says, how we are RARELY prepared. We live with assumptions that the car we drive will be okay. If it has fuel, it should go, right?

When you find yourself in a dark parking lot on a stormy night, with a smoking car and dead engine, it is terrifying! Then you call your hero Marv and his son, Steve - and hope they are home. While they aren't particularly spiritual, they arrive and see I made it to a church parking lot with the only light being a big white cross. Both have to wonder if angels work overtime - taking care of me!

So, say you read this, then set out on a journey. You drive or someone else does. Not a freak-out obsession, but just the question if the car is good to go? Honestly, this is not a daily thing. This is just maybe once a week or month, check the dang oil and radiator in older cars!

Secondly, suppose you lose your keys? This one perhaps is my WORSE nightmare fear as I have been driving. Damn key thief is always in my aura, misplacing them. Hiding keys on your car of course can make it a possibility for someone to find and steal your car, but more than likely - not. Hiding a key, having an extra in your purse. OH WAIT, if you happen to get locked out of your car, and the purse is RIGHT inside on your driver seat, smiling at you! Oooops. There are good places to hide the key. I am not going to list them here, in case a car thief is reading this because they have nothing better to do, today. Research this! Then, shhhh, have someone help you if need be. OK, so that is key on KEYS!

How about this big quantum whopper that we are so SO not prepared for. Back in the day, not too long ago, there was a thing called a phone booth. Yes, A PHONE BOOTH. You put change in, made a call and wala.

Today, most of us, I can probably say, are slaves to our cell phone or LIST at home. We aren't memorizing phone numbers anymore. I was just recently told that someone has no idea what her long-time boyfriend's phone number is! Lose your cell phone. Lose your purse, no cell. NO NUMBER. Driving or not!

So, what would it be like to write down phone numbers and also hide them somewhere? I know, it seems like someone else could find them and you just gave them a number to call. But think about it, holy crap. If you do not have a number memorized, or in a panic you go blank... is there something that can be done NOW – to survive that NOW when it gets here... if it does?

Keeping numbers in your wallet is wise. In reality, if your wallet gets lost, maybe you will give someone an opportunity to build some awesome karma, and call you or a number and you will get the wallet back. WITHOUT anything – there is no way for that to happen. Please use this chapter to take a few minutes and write these numbers down. I just did!

So, a spare key, and spare written numbers, somewhere. Even in your glove compartment where you have your auto registration. Somewhere if there is no cell phone. At least, then you can go into a home, store, or ask someone if you can use their phone... and you have a number.

This is so important.   And you, on your own, are stepping up and creating some insurance that you are okay as you get back on the road again, to life.   The car, well, life happens. The phone... a way to call someone, you can do this. Hells bells, get a tatoo of gramma's number!   ANYTHING!

In my wallet, I carry a card that I mentioned in the TBI chapter, about my condition.   So if I am pulled over for reckless driving, having troubles - the card can be scanned by cop.   Or, if I get in an accident, same thing.

All that my fingers and my heart want for you - *is* to feel safer as you bust through fear ON THE ROAD AGAIN! I really think THIS chapter can help or it wouldn't have written itself! *Thank you Marvin, my part-nerd, part genius.*

Taking a little time to PROTECT your precious self – is self-respect. Self-love. Self-care. Fog-lifting.

If you literally are just getting back on the road, behind the steering wheel and want a little extra comforting insurance, tell someone. By telling someone your destination OR (and I cannot repeat this one enough) by telling someone you hit your head... this is pro-active ways to say "FFFFFFFF--- FOG, you aint gonna dominate my life! I AM WAKING UP. Even if I go through more fog, I am also learning and growing!"

One last lil' tid bit: Carry a jug of water for the radiator and YOU, and jumper cables for the battery. AKA: coffee! Hehe. WHEW. My fingers need to go take a nap or a little drive with my hidden key and written down phone numbers. Now, the kicker: Where de heck did I hide them?

Chapter 49 - Patterned Ponies

We have galloped all over life's foggy subjects in this book.
I shall call this: Random intentional writing and poetic justice.

Raised country, so much of my philosophy is --- wait ... oh,
wow, it *just* happened. Stop. I need to include this. I know
you will relate. That is why I wrote this big monsta! For being
a songwriter who could only write one page, 3 ½ minutes... I
have definitely had diarrhea of the fingers! Ya ever tried to
spell diarrhea? Sheesh! I failed, massively. And that is where
I am going with this quickly.

 I just went to type *philosophy.* I know dang well how to
spell it.   But I did it. Total blank. Nothin. Zippo. Sat here a
starrin' at the blank space after I typed: *So much of my*
------ F f f   F ff   fulyl filllos-o-fee! Maybe it should say
full-of-us- for- a- fee.

 After all, we pay a whole lotta bucks to read, listen,
attend, watch, learn, fix up, dress up "US!"

 Fog comes in so many packages. So much is about
measuring up, hitting the mark and our philosophy of life. Even
if we cannot spell it!

 Ok, I will try this again. Raised country, so much of my
philosophy of life comes from dirt, plants ... and horses. I
think we have established that several times!   You may be
saying another "Whhhaaat?"

 Remember, this isn't a scholarly book, that reads
intellectually and makes total sense. Hey I spelled THAT ONE

RIGHT!   This author, (cool, that is fun to say: author) ...   is just writin' what comes.   If you can't track my writing... welcome to the club. TRACKING!   Never read a book - by someone who shook their melon a few times - if you want it linear and making perfect sense!

At times my brain has been like a BINGO machine. Turn, turn, turn the handle and then stop and see what letters come out! B.O.N.K.O! Hey, maybe I should start a new board game based on bonks!

Have you ever thought about phonetics?   FFFF PH-ONE-TICS. I didn't even know how to spell it. Uncle Google told me.   PH = F. Hmmm. When we are little that is how we spell. How it sounds. When we are from another country, that is how we spell. Our language is wacky. Teaching English and it's proper spelling to a child or foreigner, is all about memorizing the proper spelling because much of it doesn't make sense. What if we cannot retain this memorizing stuff? I home-schooled my daughter til 9th grade and we went through all of this.

Here's one: width, length, depth... "th" right?   How TALL is something?   Height. How much does it weigh? Weight?   What's up with that? Where did the th go? The pattern seems to be when there is an "i" in the word the "e" becomes a long A.   I'll bet, at least half of us reading this say heighth. Right? There is a point to my rambling. Or, I lost ya and you went to watch a movie!

We have to memorize *patterns* in order to learn. To function.   Anyone who survived and even thrived at any complex math knows this very well. Patterns to arrive at formulas. (Okay I lasted 2 days in algebra, so have no experience here. But I watched my daughter learn it. Oooof!)

We have rules and laws to keep things in order in our state, country, and world. All of us duckies waddlin' the same direction! It is when a few duckies go against the flow, we have some troubles.

Patterns are huge. Lab animals, monkeys, zoos, horses, trick critters and US... we are amazing. We are programmed. How to respond. How to function. How to stay alive. Think how many times a child hears: NO... when they are toddlers. I've heard mamas yelling at newborns! If we do something long enough, it becomes a pattern. It is when we DON'T fit and something in our brain doesn't retain - that we feel like the odd ball. The black sheep. The inadequate.

But if we stick with the laws, rules and patterns taught our whole lives, we should fit in pretty darn good. If we say the correct things. Get the correct job. Check the correct amount of oil in the car. Pay the correct amount on the bill... on and on and...

So then, YA BONK!

Dirt. Plants. Horses.
That right there is one very strange philosophy.

DIRT: with proper amending and/or virgin soil, can grow foods to feed ourselves and the masses.

PLANTS: left to go to seed, many will reproduce themselves. Dang, one single sunflower seed alone can produce 500 seeds. What if our thoughts were positive or negative like a sunflower seed?

HORSES: full of surprises. But pattern easily. Walk, trot, canter (lope), back up. Whoa. Giddy-up. And when treated kindly, they trust. When abused, they don't. But with time and gentleness, they will forgive, forget and re-pattern into trust. At least most.

When you read about people doing amazing things after

an injury, something shifted their pattern. Or, people that go from ill, depressed, poor – rise up and become successful, powerful energies in the world. I say that because successful and powerful are not always positive! But miracle workers of light and love... THEY ARE! And we need MORE of them!

If you put someone on a horse. Tell them to run down to the end of an arena at full speed and circle a barrel, then full-guns race back home – and they have never been on a horse or barely ridden, chances are – if the horse is "patterned" it will be stoked to blast down to that barrel and rocket back. That rider, is most likely to either fall off the ass-end of that horse, backward, or if they can stay in the saddle, go flying off the side when the horse rounds the barrel, or, over and through the ears when it blasts home and slide stops! Woohoo!

By now you are probably frowning and shaking your head with thoughts like: "This woman. She is nuts! Come on, Laurie!" I am going somewhere here... I promise. Wink! Smile! Wink!

Ever been to a rodeo or watched Barrel racing? I was a barrel racer and gamer with my horse in my teens. I have always carried the weird visual of how we take a horse from the field and pattern them for barrels. Burning it into their brain. Like us in everything we know so far.

If I took you out and put you on a horse, I would teach you some things quickly, if you wanted to race around barrels. Literally, when you turn a horse "home" from the 3rd, last barrel, I swear your lips could touch behind your head. So much power there.   So fast. And then, you have to slam on the brakes from speed so as not to go over the gate or corral fencing.   Or hit the wall. You know, *little things* like that!

In ride-horse-fast training... I would first teach you how to plant your butt in that saddle. How to hold the reins and give the horse its head so it isn't being held too high and fighting with you. They need to see where they are going.

Horses with high head or forced low-head, limit their sight. It is not natural for them.

I would show you that you have brakes in your ass. YAH. You read that right. A well-trained horse can feel every shift of your body. I would teach you how to change posture coming into a barrel. (Setting up your horse to be on the correct legs or lead, to round that barrel.) I would share how to lean, stop, hold with your thighs if your butt fails! And – CRITICAL: look where you want to go! Believe it or not, it has been proven, a horse senses that. So if you are a space cadet or no idea where you are going, you might get a horse confused. The biggest and most critical part of patterning you and your horse: you and the horse would walk, trot, lope then finally run barrels full speed.

Here is the kicker (horse punchline there) - your horse, if untrained to game, did not know the barrels before either. Pretty much, if you took ANY horse in an arena, removed the lead rope and turned them loose with 3 barrels, jumps, poles etc. – and they had never seen them before, there is a good chance they would spook, snort, fart, and dash away from those things. Slowly, they would go sniff the barrels or poles. Adjust and then ignore them. Probably lay down and roll! I can't be sure of this, but I doubt there is one horse on the planet that would naturally go out and do a pattern by themselves!

The same with a race horse. If you watch a herd of mustangs, they often have one leader, possibly the stallion or dominant mare in the front – but they are not racing to see who wins. Suffice to say, you put a bunch of Thoroughbreds on a track without a rider, highly unlikely they will walk into the tiny, scary, gate shoots that ring a loud, terrifying bell when they open - to RUN LIKE HELL in a big circle, and then, naturally race the other horses to the finish line! They are deeply patterned away from their natural instinct – into racing machines. Of course, one fall, no wins... horses often end up shot, or on trucks to slaughter – deemed a loser. Injured. Worthless. Thank GOD, if some of us can't spell or do math or keep up, this doesn't happen to us!

Plenty of horses and humans get labeled losers. Just watch any sporting event and listen to the crowd. Even tiny lil kiddos playing softball. Listen to some parents.   How can we NOT get patterned? It is everywhere.

My biggest issue was about fear of rising to high, succeeding, shining my light through my music.   The haunting was my brother accusing me of being a show-off. As a little girl with shaking knees and red face, trying to sing in front of people. Patterned ponies.   That is what we become. Fear is also a pattern. And that pattern wins and stifles our lives - A LOT! FOG. Fear Of Good – in our lives. Grrrr on FEAR.

We respond with patterns. We wake up, go to work, do our day, go to sleep - in patterns.   We believe what others believe - patterns.   We want to fit in so we slip into patterns. We ARE the patterned pony. We see the barrel of life that over the years we have ran that pattern so many times it takes a mountain of energy to shift. Or say, I AM STINKIN' SICK OF RUNNIN' BARRELS. Let me run free! Buck, kick, fart, run!

Is there anything wrong with this?   Well, I go back to the altered, fogged-in, injured brain. Patterns are busted. Fragmented. Dropped off. Gone.   What we clung to or identified with - might be gone. Our humor. Our sex appeal. Our talent. Our passion. Our sparkle. Our patience. Our speaking ability. Our math. Our reading skills. Our dreams. Our goals. Patterns... gone. Blank. Our fffffphilosophy - gone.

So there we are. Fog. All that stuff that made up who we were before a bonk, or diagnoses or major loss ... was right

335

there. Touchable. Graspable! Gone. Once again, I am not thinking about these words I am sharing right now. I am touching the keys to my computer, and giving my fingers "full rein" as you would with a horse, to run as fast as it wants. NOT controlling every word. Okay, I do have spell check, as I have mentioned. Cuz the fingers and brain do not seem to party well together. The fingers have a mind of their own!

Patterned ponies. Hmm. What does this mean? Ever heard of a horse spinning and *headin' for the barn*? We 2-legged and 4-legged, and and pretty much all creatures big and small, are patterned. Creatures of habit.

For us 2-legged, this patterning applies HUGELY to our self-confidence and how we respond emotionally. So if someone pisses you off - that has pissed you off many times, there is a good chance *pattern* will kick in and tell us "There ya go - you selfish idiot human, doing it again. Stabbing me in the back, misunderstanding me." But, if we can find a way, just a flicker of: STOP. WAIT. PAUSE. Do NOT REACT to what they say... count to 10, take a deep breath... and become aware of the whopper question: "Pattern?" Asking ourselves: *Is this the only way I know how to react? Or, what if I choose NOT to react?* Just pause ...

I ask that, because there is a great line in a Randy Travis song, that says, "They say hindsight's 20/20."

Often in hindsight, at least in my life of patterned reactions - I look back and realize there was *probably* another way to react. But, it is what it is. It got me to here. And hopefully down the road - a lesson or message was revealed. A little more growth.

My thought for my brain is - before the patterned pony in me runs like hell, with my emotions or from fear, because I see the barrels or the track of life that runs me in circles... I SHALL PAUSE. Breathe in deeply. Challenge myself to see if

I can NOT pattern. NOT react. Instead, become present as possible to the NOW. Maybe, even give thanks for this opportunity to break the pattern. WHOA. That's a biggun!

SO - there you are. Butt in the saddle. Horse's head up. Ears forward. Looking at the 3-barrel pattern waiting down in the arena. Horse's nostrils flair. You wait for your turn. Horse gets excited and starts dancing. Ready? Your heart rate quickens a bit. You have patterned for this moment for your 16 to 25 second run. Boom! You two take off full speed. Come in to the first barrel, butt planted, looking where you want to go, tucked, shifting weight, leaned, then around the barrel, straightening out to the next, leaning forward, fast as you two can go, into barrel two, tucked butt, leanin', straightening out, look where you want to go, zoom to the third... tucked, leaned and around you come, then... bring'r home full speed ahead - then slide-stop! Horse breathing heavily. Your heart racing. It was a good run, 18 seconds...

Patterns are what we are made of. Patterns how to walk, talk, spell, read, sing, create, build, think. It is when you simply become aware of this, when the thinker ball on yer shoulders is injured, altered, disappearing - THEN you understand all of this. You understand patterns get broken.

When a horse gets soured on barrel racing and gaming and no longer is calm... from all the hurry up, race, then stop - it is recommended to go on a beautiful trail ride. Calm its mind. Change patterns!

Sometimes the patterned pony in us - keeps us calm. Familiar. Sometimes it is the patterns that keep us *from* growing and keeps us *stuck* in THE FOG. So, how is yer butt. Got saddle sores? THAT was quite a writing ride! Giddy-up!

Okay so that was a butt-load on horses. You can tell where I got a lot of my ffffffphilosophy training. Farming, dirt, plants came later.

One thing farmers are learning - is all about the natural cycles, bugs, companion planting and putting natural balance back in our depleted soils.

While I do plant straight rows most the time, I also toss in wacky circles, teepees, flowers with greens, stack rocks, put out little froggy houses with bowls of water, push in old dead branches to encourage birds to come sing to me. I use my IMPERFECT PERFECTION technique to have fun and encourage healthy environments. Organic farming takes a few more little tricks to fight off daggum flea beetles that can devour precious kale and hard to get out of the soil, and all kinds of other pests... but, adding herbs, flowers and as I mentioned, companion plants, it confuses bugs.

I kinda like that! No poison. Just confusion in a good way!

Just like patterned ponies, we get stuck in ruts. We plant, we speak, we react the same way. Shake it up a bit, add some feisty or aromatic herbs to the soup pot of your life or take a horse out on a trail instead of rounding barrels. WE THE PONY, can break our patterns but first we have to become aware of them.

Again, awareness is big. Just deciding to try a different way is all it may take for you to break a pattern. Why not? Life is short. Why not try something different. Why not smile while someone is stabbing you in the back thinking, gosh, they sure are stuck in their pattern. But I am not. I am not reacting. I am smiling. Nice big, deep breath. Turning to see a bird land on a branch, or a tiny bee working hard. Or smelling the air, or, or, or...

338

WE have this in us. No matter what shape we are in. Choices. We can choose what we ingest. We can choose how we react. We can choose to use our fog as a teacher to bring us around to a more authentic us. And from there, a more positive us can emerge. When we are being real, the world benefits.

May we break patterns and run free to be who we are really meant to be!

May our souls be rich soil, to grow healthy plants of love, and.. may we be like the sunflower... reproduce many seeds of GOOD to share with the world.

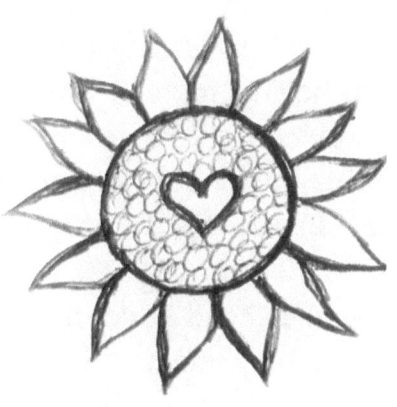

I have jumped around and probably shocked a few - in what, or how I have shared in this book of *brain*. I stand my ground in believing that we go through this stuff to learn. Learning about us, learn about our fellow humans, and how we fit.

When a person is braving up to look at a shift, of health, wealth, mental, physical or spiritual... *that* is some big stuff! Thick fog! Aside from the injury symptoms. It takes a lot of courage and energy. Sometimes we simply need to go back to bed! Not force this important growing. Other times, I think deep down, we know when we need to push through.

Finishing this book during planting season on my farm, I got this vision of hosting a big fundraiser event on the Summer Solistice for Alzheimers. With a bank account empty, energy gone, recent injuring to my hip – and inflammation back in the whole body... and trying to finish this book, I was getting BIG red flags. This is a tell-tale sign of too much. Ironically I ended up having to take Gabapentin due to some brain zapping, legs weak and blurry vision seizure episodes. As I have said, writing this book about lifting fog doesn't mean it is lifted permanently. But to try to stay present. Those zaps told me to scale back.

Presently, I have a hard time taking days off, taking care of two places and my mom. But the knowing - that CHANGE does happen, carries me. Two years ago, my dad was out mowing his lawn. Not in good shape, Dementia was present, but he was right down the road. Today, I am mowing his lawn.

Much like the black hole, if someone doesn't know that you are desperate and need help, how can they choose to step up and help? Plus, this is where the pull forth to say KEEP ON, keep farming, writing, singing, helping others - mixes me up. I need it for sanity. But I don't take much time for time to rest.   Work can be toxic. It can rule your life. Own you. I see that all the time. I heard it my whole life with my folks. Always, over-worked and under-paid. Where was the joy?

Life doesn't seem to stop and bow down to us paving a gentle, stress-free path. The work. The noise. The news. The pollution. The busy. The TOXINS.   Our country is so medicated. Trying to drug pain, depression, anxiety, insomnia, disease. When you get injured – all the above can remain. It does not go away. Now, it is your altered brain trying to fit in.

On this journey to lifting fog, toxins are a big challenge. Toxins. We have ladies who end up fighting for their lives with toxic shock syndrome from tampons. We get into cities where pollutants are belching out and we are breathing this into our beautiful lungs.   We go into hospitals and nursing homes and the water is treated so heavily with Chlorine, that even your Dementia father could smell it and tried to toss the stinky glass across the room.

Perhaps we meet someone very toxic, who is so into you, and soon - you find they are a cling-on. Or the other way around. You - become obsessed with them! We may not know what to do with that person. Or we obsess with the past toxic thoughts of anger and resentment. Perhaps we go to the store and bring home toxic hair supplies, laundry soaps, nail polishes, spray paints, colognes, perfumes, air fresheners, shower cleaners, and on and on and fill our homes with toxins.

Then there is foods and drink. The chemicals. The pesticide sprays. The hormones. The cupboards full of long-shelf life, just-add-water, fast foods.   Hey, I know. I LOVE my once-in-awhile MAC 'n CHEESE! Dang it! or my frozen burrito. My can of cream of mushroom soup with MSG.   In moderation of course... cuz my fingers swell!

I could never walk into a home with new carpet or strong paint smells.   My mom has a habit of painting her fingernails with toxic polish, with her bedroom door closed and no clue - then gets offended if I say anything. My dad use to start his chainsaw inside a barn and suck in all that exhaust. Then come out dazed and confused, and blame mom!

Some folk aren't aware of certain candles or diffusers that are very toxic. Aromatic toxins! Who'da thunk! Traffic belches out exhaust. People belch out their emotions.

Toxic obsession about pain is a doozy.   To listen to someone's some-total of their day or present life: "Which pain pill, or this happened, or oh my pain!"   It is their toxic pattern that suddenly can become *yours*.   If you are not strong going in to this, which most of us aren't. We somehow have to find that toxic-free orb to live in or we absorb all that stuff into our system as well. With or without brain injury!

Some people do a fell swoop cleaning. They look around their house.   If they SMELL the bleach, perfumes, soap, dryer sheet, comet, hair soap, hair spray, deodorants. Shoot, even most flea collars and kitty litter have chemicals.   They decide: if I can smell this, it is gone. Well, hopefully not the kitty. Hopefully better products!   Some even take out all plastic that might be out- gassing. Others may not have that luxury. It may be those you live with who insist on the STINK! Meanwhile, their actions, their patterns give you headaches, lungs burn, dizzy spells.

I went to a movie by myself one night. The place was full. Found one seat not too close to the screen, so I took it.

About 15 minutes into the movie, my lungs began to burn. A woman was snuggling with her partner to the left of me. She smiled when I sat down. But when she sat straight up, I realized it was her. Her PERFUME. Omgosh! Strong. Sweet. Burning. By then the place was packed - so I had to tolerate the smell or leave. By the time the movie was over, my head felt like I had a shot of whiskey and my lungs felt like I had eaten razor blades. CRAZY stuff, all because of a woman who sprayed herself to smell PURDY! Crazy huh? I know women who wear perfume to the hospital!

I have a cousin who cannot go outside when folks are burning their wood stoves. She can't breathe. When you are injured and ill, all this stuff is amplified.

So you either lock yourself in a room - free of toxins or try to figure out how to adapt. But if the reaction is worse than the social potential, you may have to just protect yourself. The kicker of it all, is... that WE may be the toxic one. If we are obsessed with our condition and/or... frankly, TOXINS!

HA! By now, you are probably going cross-eyed and asking, "Laurie, who is on first, what is on second? Round and around!" All of this is about *awareness*. Others, ourselves. Even in tiny bite-size thoughts - that show us our surroundings, our patterns, and what we can and cannot change. Toxins come in our thoughts too. Anger, blame, gossip. Obsessions over who we think is worthy, not worthy, should burn in hell, or receive heavenly blessings. Obsessed thinking comes to many, not just the brain injured.

In toxic dramatic company, you have to be careful how quickly you can get sucked in and dampen your, perhaps already worn-out soul, or see that they are not the bad guy or gal. They are just living in their toxic loop. But given too much time together, the loop might include you.

I have to look at my OWN loop of thoughts. My own toxins.

The altered brain does have a tendency, while in survival mode, to get stuck in a toxic loop. Looking at toxins it is just one more thing as we lift fog, in our tool box of healing.

All this stuff does not come with a manual. Toxic is toxic. Our challenge is to find some balance. If you do live with a toxic person, and it might be a child or elderly that cannot be kicked out on their ears, then the answer might be: create a NON-toxic space in your home. Deep breathing. Go outside. Special walks. Corners. Mantels. Meditation. Books. Music. Warm bath. Stretching. Some *TLC for your san-i-ty!*

I cannot forget to mention one big toxin that has control over our society... besides sugars and MSG food enhancements that make us CRAVE more... for many it is the obsessive use of a computer and/or cell phones... texting and social media. My oh my.

Another is the television. As I mentioned before. Waking up to what we dump into our system, via movies, news... if the media is doing their job well, we will get hooked. Pulled in. The drama. The update. The story. The political angle and so on. Just like the cork or the cap on the liqueur, or pill bottle - the TV comes with the POWER button. A lot of people seem to need the white noise for company leaving the TV on because silence is too lonely. Having my mom living here, with morning news, talk TV and evening shows, my house has felt like it shrunk. Thank goodness, honestly, that I could go in my back room and type these words about toxins!

Lifting fog, it comes back to asking: WHAT CAN I DO WITH THIS – NOW? How can I help myself heal?

Funny how fear will appear in the tiniest cracks. Getting closer to finishing this book, I watched a story on TV about a man and his wife. He had been attacked, his brain split open with a steel pipe, and had to learn everything over again, including breathing. His wife wrote a book about their journey.

In that moment, seeing that, with a recent hit to my head by a steel bar that fell from the ceiling, I just sat that there. I had just typed about toxins.   I was silent. I walked in my office and looked at the laptop where this book is held.

The fear thought was: I am so much better off than what happened to that man. My life did not change THAT much. Gosh. What the hell am I doing writing a book?   Should I pick up the laptop, take it to the river bridge and toss it in? Let go of this notion that I can help another?

I typed those words because I wanted you to read how this mind can work. As can anyone's. Especially injured. Fogged. From this, here is what wants to be written: I end this chapter with the biggest toxin of all that can kill our lives or limit us from living a full life: FEAR.

Even having the courage to stop or avoid all the other toxins, fear can take over.   Or, by clearing our bodies, minds, spirits, here's an even biggy'r: WE FEAR WE WILL GET ALL THE TOXINS OUT OF THE WAY... and then, we will be forced to live a full life BECAUSE we are healed. No drama. No excuse for not being our whole self.   BE BRAVE. Lean in to this. Honor your fear - then choose to say, "NO MORE - FEAR! NO MORE will you toxic-ally own my life. I can do this."

I said it right here in real time, that I *could* take my book and throw it in the river. Let go. Give up. OR... push through the FOG... and GO FOR IT!

I 'spose if you just read that last sentence,
FEAR did NOT win! Woohoosky!

Chapter 51 – Brain Soup, Ya Gotta Poop!

If by chance you did not have a brain injury going into reading my book, and did not know squat about fog, I am surmisin' here that by now, your brain is feeling a smidgin' swirly - to follow along with this writing. The real funny is ... if you do not know me, you do not know if I may have attended college with off-the-chart-grades and graduated with journalism and English Lit as my majors. I shall not reveal. Hey, if you are laughing - it IS possible I am just yankin' yer chain and all this writing is, as my daddy profoundly labeled: horseshit!

Or, you get this book. This journey. I hope you feel like we had a great visit. You have been at my house or me at yours, and we have talked. Left our damn cell phones in the car. We related. Cried. Laughed. Drank too much coffee or ate too much dark chocolate. Something nice!

So then of course we must ask ourselves, "Self, why is Laurie calling this Brain soup, ya gotta poop? Funny, I am asking the same dang thangy. In reality, til my fingers hit the keys, like paint on a white canvas, I never know what will come out. Just like songwriting. My muse, my angels, spirit, love, God, whatever helps me... I just say thanks and write on. It has something to do with de-toxing all that stuff from the previous chapter.

So here is what my fingers want to say: Ya gotta poop! Literally and mentally. Ya gotta let it out. Ya gotta NOT get constipated and obsessed with YOU. Your condition. You won't lift a bit of fog if you sit on the pot of life all day, and don't try.

I have mentioned before that we have to choose what we digest and put into our heads and bodies. If you are a heavy carb hog and pig on breads, eat tons of proteins, and never take in fiber to break it up and send her down the tube... yer gonna sit on the pot of life for a long time! PLUGGED UP TIGHT!

Okay, I had to just stop and have a *giggle talk* with my fingers!

I'm back. Hydrating your body is the best medicine you can do. You cannot drink enough plaino jaino water. It's crazy. But we don't. I have a friend who just went on a water fast. I was shaking my head. NO WAY. How can someone live on water. I watched my dad die without food and little water. But it was quantity. Dad's body was checking out. Water fasting is about cleansing. My friend was doing this fast to purge his system of all the stuff stuck in his cells. The sugars. The proteins. The fats. All that circled around and messed with his digestion. He swore that plain water – was it.

Now, I am not convinced this body is going to do such a fast. One 2-day purging colon-osto-poo at 50, was enough to say, no, I like food. But it is learning that it is WHAT we eat. A break of food can be beneficial. Many people do a one-day fast, weekly or monthly.

So that is the food part. Then, there is WHAT we think. Brain input. A person might do all that fasting and find out the indigestion was literally reducing something from their diet. Beer, sugar, white flours, corn, or ... constipating thoughts! Stress. ANXIETY. Remember the patterned pony? We don't start out full of this. We become patterns.

347

Breaking them and becoming aware and present - breaks patterns up and helps lift fog to a CLEARER version of US.

Babies eat, babies poop. Eat. Poop. Repeat. A lot. There food goes through, serves the body and moves on. Our food, if it is constipating, hangs out in that extremely long intestinal journey from mouth to butt and can reek havoc. Gas, Irritable bowel syndrome, pain, constipation, inflammation, cancer... all because we GET STUCK.

SO, POOP SOUP. When you decide to clean out your system to the best you can while you are fogged in or coming out of the fog and truly wanting to be a new clearer version of yourself... there is some detoxing required BODY, MIND and SPIRIT, if you believe in spirit. The first two are proven. Just look in the mirror!

Certain foods are terrific for detoxing. It is known the herb, Milk Thistle, is amazing for detoxing the liver where all the nasty stuff we consume, including medicines, has to go through. Certain foods can also blast things apart and help cleanse and detox.

Good ol' cabbage is one of them. Any greens that you enjoy. Carrots if you aren't a diabetic with the sugar levels, are wonderful. But rather than give you all that info that is already out there – I would just like to leave you with a recipe for literal POOP SOUP.
Two actually:

Literally, a good cabbage, chicken or vege broth soup with carrots, onions, cauliflower, kale, celery, garlic, sea salt, black pepper, some ginger, parsley and tossing in some brown rice... this is a favorite detox soup. If you can handle heat, a little cayenne helps do some cookin' too.

Detoxing a plugged-up brain and thoughts aka fog – is a little more complicated.

A brain soup is any input to your brain that is calming. Positive. Quieting the noise. The busy Monkey mind. One is Meditation. This can be very challenging. I know. I have busy Betty brain - often. So when I get really quiet and try to meditate, I often end up making my grocery list instead of OHMing and deciding I have to pee instead of peace out.

So here is a tip: Give thanks. If you cannot get totally quiet and go within, blocking out your patterns, the noise, the lists, the grudges... if you can just take a few minutes throughout the day, pause, (shoot, even set a timer if you have to) and take in a deep breath and simply say, THANK YOU.. as you exhale..

Oh my gosh, it is amazing how clearing constipated thinking in life - can suddenly shift into a blessing. Again... Deep breath. THANK YOU - as you breathe out. Repeat. And ya know what, it is your secret poop soup. The world can be pounding down around you. NEWS at 5. Politics blah blah. Family drama. Work overload. Lack of money. Bills due. But in that little moment that NO ONE can take away from you, you can intentionally ingest a sip, or a bowl, of *soul poop soup*. YOU HAVE CONTROL!   This can DETOX your thoughts, your perspective and help lift fog.   You do this, drink water, stay hydrated, eat well, toss in some stretches to move the organs, let go of fear... hot doggies... look out FOG! I'll be seeing your story, NEWS at 5!

OK, so there ya go. Fingers just gave me a THUMBS UP. I am chuckling. Breathing in. Saying thanks, breathing out. Gnawing on a carrot, drinking some water, and gonna stretch. Then head back to my padded cell! Hehehe!

Hmmm,
Probably need a little poem
of how we need to poop -
get rid of crappy thoughts and stuff
that bubbles 'round like soup.

Festering all the good stuff
that is 'spose to help our mind -
need to unload life's toxic gunk
and get on with our lives.

So maybe I didn't just hit my head
to fog up and hurt my brain -
maybe this is opportunity
to start all over again.

I might be constipated
maybe that's why I hit -
so I will attempt to lift this fog -
by taking a life good _____!

Ha. Bet you thought I was going to type
shit. Nah, I'll let you imagine...

I am so... my father's daughter. Bahaha!
LLL

350

Chapter 52 - Holy Cowbells! A buried treasure!

I was just about to say adios and something made me go to my old OLD computer. Looking for lyrics to a song, I see a file that says: WHEN THE FOG LIFTS. Huh? I open it. Whoa! There, lookin' back at me, is this writing below, that I had written just 2 months after my FIRST nasty concussion. 2008!

While I have said most of this already throughout this book, this was written to give to a neurologist early on. To try to describe, best I could, this bizarre new ME. So, here we are one chapter before the end. And I found THIS writing. My gut says SHARE IT! I think it is a MEANT TO BE.

Maybe YOU will write your own journal or book, partially inspired by my ballsy, unconventional, honest efforts to share. I hope so. I will read it! YOU are a teacher. Just by showing up and living! Whatever you are going through, you ... can touch another person's life.

'From holes to whole' an entry for a some day "aha" book:
When the Fog Lifts
Written: September 9, 2008

Laurie Lee Lewis

Date of head injury July 17th. Hit right side of head really hard on steel hanging lamp. Goose egg bump and severe pain in left side of neck.

Week 1

Besides a headache and lump the first 2 days were fairly normal.

The 19th I began feeling sick. Flu-like symptoms. I noted my eyelids swelled for nearly the first week. Headaches kept coming and going. I could not sleep. The temperature was in the 90's and I could not handle it at all. I had had a bad heat stroke 2 years prior and felt some of the same symptoms.

2 weeks passed and I seemed to be getting worse neurologically. The foggy flu and achy pains and dizzies moved into disoriented, ears began ringing, a hot oil feeling in my left side of my head constantly. I found myself doing weird stuff like sitting outside to pull a weed and instead laying my head down on the grass. I would start to walk outside and not sure what I was doing. Tipping over to the left.

End of Week 2

I finally went to Dr. H.. Still headaches and not sleeping well. So tired and much pain in my back/neck. She thought it was inner ear but did not suggest anything to help me other than it needed to run its course. I did not remember that I had hit my head. Just was puzzled that I felt so bad. Walking and driving was so hard but I continued to drive. I felt drunk and fogged in. I had to write things down over and over. No energy. The same woman who was slinging a pick ax and ripping up weeds the month prior and even performing music on stage! Who was I now?

I tried to tug o war with our dog and one jerk totally sent me of kilter and I realized how totally week I was. I also noticed that I could not type very well. My words were either all there but backward or a bunch of garble. Still are -when I get tired. Not hearing my music anymore confirmed something serious.

Week 3
Ringing in ears worsened. I went to my chiropractor. His adjustment seemed to worsen the headaches. After a few more days, Dr H. suggested I go to the walk in after hours to see a Dr. Dr. G. asked me soon after I told him my symptoms if I had hit my head? Hmmm. I had to think. Then, I remembered hitting it so hard it put me to the ground. G. thought it was a concussion and explained why the pain/injury was on my left side rather than my right where I hit. He did some neurological testing. The florescent lights were horrible. Dr G. ordered an MRI for the following week. And did suggest if it was inner ear, that I should do saline rinses. I did. No help.

Week 3 and $\frac{1}{2}$.
After the MRI New symptoms followed. I drove myself to the MRI and did not use any meds. I felt stoned already. I had such a terrible headache driving home that I felt I barely made it.
As the week progressed, sure I was getting better or wanted to be better,
I tried to mow the law. I even wore an air mask so as not to ingest fumes. I had to shut off the mower and found myself drenched, shaking and barely getting into the house after only a bit of exertion. My legs were jerking. It was the first time I wondered if I had some type of disease. MS or Parkinsons. My walking and tipping was worse. My typing got worse.

Week 4

The MRI tests and blood tests Dr H. had taken were good. I canceled events, hesitated going anywhere with my family that was busy.

We went camping and I found myself pouring through health books trying to find what might lift the fog. Dr. Hutchinson had prescribed massage. I had 2. Both were hard to drive to and from. My memory and speech was altered. I found I was constantly searching for words I knew but could not recall for my sentences. I would forget something immediately.

Week 5
We went camping again very close by. I drove our car back home because I did not pack very well. Forget nearly everything. Driving to and from was like I was dreaming and drunk. Everything I did had a glaze of slowness, to think, to process, to answer. In some ways I tried to see this as a blessing so I would not over stress over details. My family was not use to this laid back person. But in reality I was struggling.
One day I got mad and grabbed a shovel and pick ax and started chopping out grass for a flower bed. I found myself grunting and chopping in a labored manner. I felt mad and wanted to cry at this weak person.
That night, shocks went through the base of my skull nearly all night, the hot oil feeling that was there constantly was worse. No sleep did not help my condition.

Week 6
I called the DR again insisting more blood or something be taken.
Both H. and G. had concluded their diagnosis that I was in

354

post concussion faze. Not much advice. Only what I could find on the internet.

This week I drove to Bham with my daughter. We did only a few things and I knew I needed to get home. Dizzy, lightheaded, weak. Driving home, I had to keep asking myself who was driving, how fast was I going and why did I not associate my foot to the speed. This was the last driving I did to Bellingham!

Also that week, walking back in from taking garbage cans out to the street, the sun was shining on my head. Within minutes I felt a wave a white and fell to the ground. I tried to stand and the white returned. I called for my daughter and hung onto her as we went back in the house.

That weekend, trying to help my husband outside a bit, I found most of the time was standing, spaced out. I cried once, feeling so lost and useless.

Week 7

I got into an ear nose and throat Dr. My husband took me. The carpet had a pattern on it which kept tipping me over. The lights were bright. Dr. shut them off. He did not see any infection. Said the MRI was good. Did a hearing test and noted loss in high end of left ear. My comment was I could not hear passed "Tinkerbell's high pitch ringing" ie same tone.

He agreed that I had a concussion and time was my healer.

This whole week my head felt swelled and tight. I told my daughter I wanted to cut all my hair off very short.

Week 8.

That Monday /Sept. Tues. 1st and 2nd I felt a bit better. I recognized something in the mirror. Me! I remember the sense of I KNOW YOU. You are the face that disappeared about 8 weeks ago. I also noticed I was walking faster. Not fast, but without having to think about each step. Wow. We had purchased new chickens and they needed a shelter lean-to. My hubby did not have time and I love to build. So I decided to try. I used the hammer and a small saw.

Though I was still speaking slowly, thinking and forgetting a lot, I felt some accomplishments by cobbling together this thing. I did not sleep well. More skull shocks the first night. But I felt kinda ok and was not done the next day so I continued. Tuesday night was horrible. I fogged out, could barely keep a sentence straight, stood and starred a fair bit. Felt weepy. Wed. my dad drove me for more blood tests that I insisted Dr. Hutchinson order. Look for something off. Neurological diseases. Something. Blood work came back ok. Friday the 5th my hubby drove my to the Chiropractor for another stab at my neck. I did not feel well. He adjusted. Wes and daughter Callie went to a toy store 3 blocks down in Fairhaven. I called when I was done. Said I think I could walk. It would be good for me. I was wrong. A block down, I noticed I disassociated with my feet taking steps as if I were floating. Scary. As I got to the second block, I noticed that every brick, windowpane, doorway, cobblestone, anything with a straight line was amplified. I felt as if they were swallowing me. I seemed to be losing my common sense to call Wes. I kept stopping. Bracing myself. Trying to find something without damn lines.

At the last cross street, I must have looked drunk. I could not tell if I was moving forward or backward. I spotted a ROUNDED bike rack and clung to it as I gathered my balance. I could have called Wes but was angry that I could not fix this. I only had to walk across one more cobbled road. I took a deep breath and headed across. It was about half way that I honestly was not sure I would stay upright any longer. I wanted to drop to my knees and crawl. I was so scared. I finally got to the door of the store. Walked in. Spotted Wes' back. Did not even get his attention. I spotted a ROUND wooden table and immediately made my way over to it. Sat and looked down. All the stimuli in the store was making me swirl. My daughter saw me and came up to show me something. I wanted to burst into tears. Wes saw me and came to give me the keys so I could head to the truck. I looked up and had such pain in my eyes he knew that was impossible. When he helped me to the truck I got in and began to sob. I could not hold it in anymore. That night I felt very bad. Not sleeping well. Speaking with spaces. Pretty crummy. The weekend was slow and I did not do much.

Week 9
Monday, headache, typing badly, vision blurry. Vision has been blurry all along. But worsens at different times of the day. Same as ringing in the ears.
I can read, but not for long. It is distance that is so blurry. WE are again trying to get ready for a camp trip this weekend and I have had to write things down. I noted that when I type lists in bold ariel I could process my notes better than my hand writing. I continue to worry that I am burning food on the stove, or leaving the bathtub running or (like today) overflowing the kitchen sink, forgetting soap in the washer, wonder what I am doing. My head still feels tight about 90% of the time. And the headaches come in double places at times. The place I hit it and the left side.

Today, Tuesday the 9th I had a window this morning of about 1 hour, as I made the bed and puttered that I felt lighter, more like me, before the fog moved in.
Throughout this whole 9 weeks there have been

hours/clusters where I have felt this. One unusual awareness I had, a couple times over the past 9 weeks was when I had a little wine and a couple beers, different times. I was aware that I could not feel the alcohol, rather I felt less frustrated. Meaning I felt the buzz all the time and want to sober up, but so far, I have not.

I did, out of stubbornness, drive my little girl to the local store a few miles away at about 40 mph last week, just to get a cup of coffee and do something sort of normal. I was exhausted to get home. But it was fun too. The slowness has made me try to just take one moment at a time. Which I suppose we all need at times in our busy lives. I also noticed I have drunk more coffee that normal, desperate to clear the fog, to no avail.

This past week I felt more depressed and angry. When I heard my husband tell someone on the phone that his wife had a mild concussion and has been experiencing some mild symptoms, it bothered me. He meant no harm, it was just my perception.

Trying to figure out how I am going to home school Callie for 5th grade has been strange. But some of this space actually has slowed me to focus on more detail. Clutter has been the worst poison and too much activity.

I have done the best, in a quiet setting, in my yard, sitting and pulling a week and being close to earth. My garden has brought both frustration, over all the weeds that weren't there in June and it has brought some peace that it grew without me and turned out beautiful.

The city, loud noises, talking on the phones, bright lights and too many faces causes me to feel dizzy. Too many people talking at once tosses me to a swirls place. I have a strange disconnect to my body's thermostat too. When everyone is hot I might be into chills. When others are cold I might be in a t shirt. When I cook I have to be careful not to burn me. I don't seem to feel the first second or two that protects us. Same with frozen stuff.

As the ear Dr. said, "time is my medicine now" I imagine that is true, while the holes heal and I find wholeness again, I hope. I think time has a mind of its own!

I went to bed.
A *happy* head -
The next day ...
shampoo'd away

A lamp of steel
made life *surreal* -
No more play ...
shampooer put away.

Doctor please
what's *happened* to me -
Fog rolled in ...
will it lift again?

Don't you see
this *aint* me -
a slippery slope ...
Please give me hope.

LLL

Chapter 53 - Thy will be done

When I was little, I always wondered what a THY was. I knew what a thigh was. I knew what a Sty was. But the whole Thy and God mixture just didn't compute.

Now this book obviously did not stick to some rigid rules of writing. Grammar and punctuation were the raw, un-polished version, like me. After all, if I was to try to speak, as if we were in a coffee shop yappin' about brain injury – well I would not speak like we write, like this: So (comma) you say you hit your head (question mark) That must have been horrible (exclamation mark.)

Right? So to write this book, without reservation, without worrying that I would not hit the professional writer mark to appease a certain intelligent audience, I just wrote. And wrote! And wrote some more!

So what the heck does THY WILL BE DONE have anything to do with WHEN THE FOG LIFTS, or F.O.G. = FEAR OF GOD/GOOD or FAITH OF GOD/GOOD and mostly... TBI/brain injury/concussion/multiple concussions?

Well, since you asked, I decided to ask Uncle Google what he thought about the word THY. To my surprise, it did not mean what I thought. It wasn't God or father or holiness. It was more about yourself, your, you.   Huh? You will be done? Yourself will be done? Your will – be done?

Honestly, this was not how I thought I would walk away from our time together. Many chapters have been me just placing my fingers on the keys and lettin'r rip.

I think my whole heart and soul wants to leave with you a huge *thank you*.   One for being courageous enough to want to read a woman's long-winded journey through so many concussions. Furthermore, to even consider believing me.

Secondly, from whichever viewpoint you are coming from - the injured, the caregiver, the loved-one, sibling, friend, lover, teacher, doctor ... this world is fast. This world is hard to keep up with. We all know that. Injured brains "our computer" makes the world seem faster and we seem - *so much* slower. To keep up - without *giving up*, is the hardest part to explain. The fine line of thriving and barely surviving- can walk side by side on any given day. In other words, we need to have a little more grace with each other. We do not walk in another's shoes. Or carry around *their* brain. *Their* life.

You can start out a day fogged-over and not want to be here, yet end the same day, with clarity and an unimaginable sense of ever wanting life to end.   Or vice verse.

No wonder doctors trying to help their post-concussion patients have a little bit of helpless or even a dumb-founded look on their face, knowing *they* really cannot *heal* us.

They can maybe put a band-aid of medicine on us via sleep aids, pain med, anti-depressants, anti-seizure, anti-anxiety meds... (to ease the discomfort and help us cope) but in reality, most of the time, *TIME* is the ultimate healing medicine. So let's see if I get what my fingers are trying to tell me and you, before we say goodbye:

THY WILL BE DONE. Who? What? God? Us? Both? The highest good, in some wacky way, will be done? I injured my brain for my soul growth? For others around me? My own deep core knowing that I was suppose to go through this for a reason? And, if I pay attention as I heal, try to be grateful and grow, then - THEN... THY *FOG* will be done? Aka, MY

FOG - in time WILL lift and BE DONE? Whoa! That really blew my fingers away to write!

Whether the brain heals completely, rebuilds cells, awakens your genius or compassion, takes you to the depth of the black hole, helps you forgive and forget, deepens your sense of life's gift of giving and connectedness, busts open a spiritual awakening and purpose – I don't know. But I do know that we can choose to be open to unlimited possibilities! Again and again.

The fact that you are reading a book, that I threw away several times and told God there was no way this brain could write it. To me, this says HOPE is alive, deep inside of us, even when we are fogged completely over. I wanted to write. Just didn't know how. I wanted to sound well-researched and fully healed, then write. Ah, not! Just one letter typed after another. Which, turned into a dag gum epic qua-trilogy thang!

Hope and time, partnered together – can lift fog. If you get that much from this book, Thy *Will* Be Done. YUP. Thy done wrote this book. THANK YOU GOD! You had a pretty stubborn kid that made spell check work very hard!

We have much more input – than we realize. If fog forces us to slow down, pay attention, try to take off the masks we wear to be approved of, perhaps wear the idea that we are spirits here on earth, signed up for a human experience. Perhaps when fog rolls in, it is a sign that we have forgotten, so try to honor the fog as a teacher and reminder. Try to deeply breathe in your worthiness. Ultimately, bust through fear, and WHEN THE FOG LIFTS, on even the littlest shifts and awakening - remember to be grateful. That = happiness/peace.

This kinda tripped me out writing such a mongo-size book. I hope to heck that I made some sense! Time for this singing farmer to grow food to feed the hungry and, sing!

And the Oscar goes to: All who face the fog, and are brave enough to say, **"SHOW ME and THY WILL BE DONE!" LIFT FOG LIFT!**

My own Oscar award goes to THUMPER the styrofoam head, beaming with an aura of over 20 pokey toothpicks ... reminding me of my journey... and the new chapters ahead.

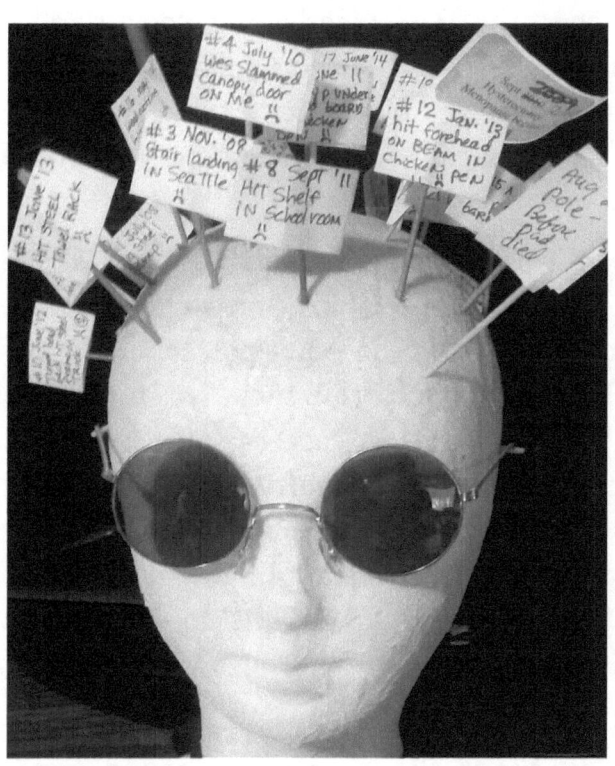

Chapter 54: Head, Heart, Hands, Health

Wait! Hold it! I am not quite done.

Ah, pig turds. I thought that last chapter was going to be my elegant sign off and ride into the THY WILL BE DONE, sunset. I hoped that I inspired you in some small way, to take care of yourself on this journey called life. As I typed the last words, deep down, I felt something was chewin' on my belly, sayin' "Uh, Laurie, NOT quite done yet. Put your fingers back on the keys and type."

My goal was to share something that would offer you HOPE on your journey.   I shared how even though I have one mighty scarred *HEAD*, from multiple concussions, bumps and thumps, I keep trying to think, write and share good thoughts. I have tried to use my *HEART* to show love, kindness, forgiveness and loyalty. I have tried to use my *HANDS* to write, record and perform positive songs for the world and grow healthy foods for the hungry. And, I have tried to believe that my *HEALTH* is an on-going reflection of how I am doing in life. Trying always, to learn, heal and grow stronger to serve humanity.

With all those thoughts – I realized something VERY profound ... and *this* is what popped into my head:

When I was Laurie Little, rather, *little* Laurie Little, I had a Shetland pony named Silver. I grew up on the farm that

I now farm myself. Farming was a magical life, all about work ethics and doing your part.

I was in 4-H for years. Our club was called: Swift Kicks. Gotta few of those in my time! We were a motley little bunch of low-income kiddos, who learned about self-esteem, being a team player and horses! Ironically, though desperately shy, I somehow was voted 4-H president, 2 years in a row, after I got my big "best friend" quarter horse, Wrambler. It befuddled me that kids looked to me as a leader. I 'spose God was starting to show me something. (I even came across my leadership ring!) It's ancient now!

I went on to ride many horses, professionally model, did TV and radio commercials, toured as a country singer-songwriter, produced 12 CDs, and finally returned to the farm - to raise my daughter.

In writing this last chapter, I realized that while I forget what I had for breakfast, or if I even ate - I never forgot the pledge that we kiddos all took as 4-H members:

"I pledge my HEAD to clearer thinking, My HEART to greater loyalty, My HANDS to larger service, My HEALTH to better living, for my club, my community, my country and my world. (Permission granted by the USDA 4-H National Headquarters) Thank you!

This got my curiosity up about 4-H's history and what it is doing today and this is what I found out:

What was founded in 1902, is now a global youth organization inspiring young people to reach for their full potential! Wow! To any parent reading this that might like their child to get involved, I highly recommend contacting your local 4-H club or extension office. Or http://4-h.org They love parents too!

I think *that* pledge has been subconsciously guiding me the past 40 years! Holy Moly! Pretty dang cool! Only discovered because of this book! The 4-H pledge actually describes our potential to build a better world by striving to live a value-filled life. When we truly wake up to gratitude and **One world, One family** connectedness ... *that* is WHEN THE FOG LIFTS. It is NOT us and them. IT IS ALL **US**.

Imagine *if* our world leaders would pledge this as well! Imagine if our Presidents had to go through 4-H and learn about team players. All for one. Okay, I just had to put that in there. 'Tis my book after all. But I hope I get a couple smiles from 4-Hers that remember this too!

When you are trapped in the fog in day to day life, this community idea may not appeal to you. It may stress you. NOT the intention of my writings. But head, heart, hands and health put together, can lift fog, whether you were/are in 4-H or not! It sets us back on the track of life - with purpose.

So here's a cheer to **lifting fog** that has socked in and closed dreams, love, hope, healing, spontaneity, communication, trust and truth.

So that's it. I feel kinda emotional to say goodbye. GOSH. HUG HUG HUG HUG HUG HUG HUG HUG HUG!

To lift my spirits from saying goodbye to you, I pretended that the TODAY show or Seattle King 5 TV called and asked me on for an interview. Helping me, bringing hope to others going through fog. When they asked me the big colossal question: "Laurie, what would you say fog REALLY taught you during this 10-year journey and how do you use it today?" I took a big breath, and said, "Well, I really believe, that LIFE is a GIFT. All the head injuries showed me how I went into

366

2008 very insecure. Doubting my self-worth, and *way* too worried about what other people thought."

I would pause, then I would add with a big ol' smile:

"F.O.G. Can mean: A life **FULL * OF * GOOD, FANTASTIC * OUTRAGEOUS * GOOD,** *once we recognize it as a teacher/reminder and lift the* **FEAR OF GOOD** *or* **GOD**"

A decision only we make. A conviction to our soul.

To LIVE with gratitude no matter what comes at us. To CHOOSE to ask what gift is in this fog. To SHOW ME. I WANT TO LEARN and GROW. Ultimately, **LOVE** is the greatest fog-lifter tool we have. Unconditional Love. Oh, then I would get up and sing them a pretty song! And we would hug, heart to heart! (The name of my farm.)

I have carried this knowledge and experiences painfully for 10 years. Many moments where I could not even turn on a computer. Or look at a screen. Moments when I wondered if tomorrow would come. None of us know that part of "next." But we have NOW. This big, beautiful NOW. Shoot, I could have told you all that in 2 pages, but then we would not have gotten to hang out together all this time!

Sitting in the doctor's office in Nov. 2018, in a fog of *grief* after losing my dad 3 months earlier, the doctor, who had also lost his dad to Dementia in a facility - knew my pain and said to me: "Take your pain, Laurie, and use it as inspiration."

That night, with my dad's guitar, I wrote the deepest song of my life called: THIN VEIL. Asking all about life. Pain. Missing our loved ones. Being honest about our pain. The doctor was right. I took the pain of 10 years and wrote this book. I hope it inspires.   Thank you for reading.

To end on a funny... to quote Porky Pig, (to whom I could relate very well, when I stuttered, following one concussion):
"Abadee, abadee, aah, that's all folks!"

****

I do not apologize,

for who I am today -

the scars are my life's road map,
showing me the way -

I've lived a bumpy life,
some profound, some horse shit -
but here I am now,
this book, these words, this is it.

My wake-up call, done woke me up,
words of truth I share -
I lived the fog, I know it well,
I share, because I CARE.

So take it with a grain of salt,
or believe me when I say -
live, laugh, love and learn,
before life goes away.

Big love and heart hugs.

Love, Laurie

I did it, dad. I finished the book! Thank you for helping me.
Now go sing some country music with the angels. I love you.

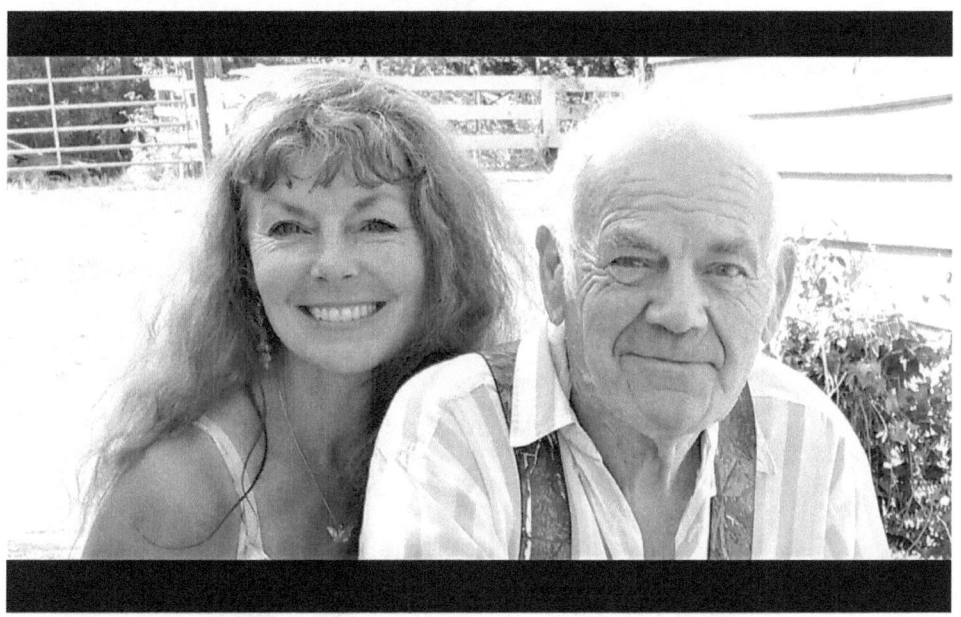

I have used lines to several of my songs throughout this book.

If you are interested in hearing or purchasing my music, I
have most of my music up on CD baby for download or actual
CDs. At: www.cdbaby.com/laurieleelewis and will be adding
more, especially when SPIRIT PLAYING HUMAN gets done.

I have several music videos up as well from my 30-year music
career on youtube: www.youtube.com/laurieleelewis

Also, if you have a gathering in which you feel my story and/or
music could contribute, I would enjoy talking to you about
that. Shoot me an email at: hearttoheartfarm@gmail.com I
am caregiver to my mom, and still farming, but hey, make me
an offer I cannot refuse. You know, some tropical cabana in
Maui or B & B in Ireland. Heck, I'll bring my daughter and
guitars and throw in a concert too! I could use the fun! visit
My website: www.hearttoheartfarm.com

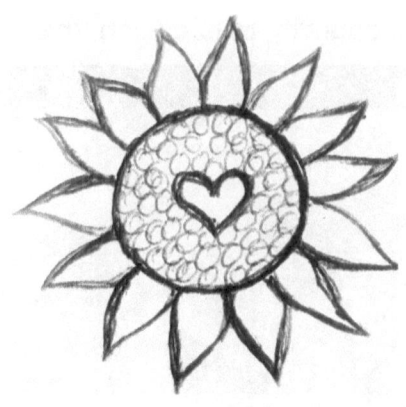

Be like the sunflower ...
stand tall, produce seeds -
leave behind in this world
heart-based thoughts - to feed.

Be like the sunflower ...
grow, learn, share -
We are the world's hope and shift
unfold your life with care.

From my heart to yours,
Love, Laurie
My farm and Life Motto:
Grow To Give, Give To Grow.